AF440447

Colorectal Cancer
in Clinical Practice

Colorectal Cancer
in Clinical Practice

Prevention, Early Detection and Management

Paul Rozen, MD
Department of Gastroenterology, Tel Aviv Sourasky Medical Center,
Tel Aviv, Israel

Graeme P Young, MD
Gastrointestinal Services, Flinders Medical Centre,
Adelaide, South Australia

Bernard Levin, MD
Division of Cancer Prevention, MD Anderson Cancer Center,
Houston, TX, USA

Stephen J Spann, MD
Department of Family and Community Medicine,
Baylor College of Medicine, Houston, TX, USA

MARTIN DUNITZ

Although every effort has been made to ensure that all owners of copyright material have been acknowledged in this publication, we would be glad to acknowledge in subsequent reprints or editions any omissions brought to our attention.

First published in the United Kingdom in 2002
by Martin Dunitz Ltd, The Livery House, 7–9 Pratt Street, London NW1 0AE

Tel.: +44(0) 20 74822202
Fax.: +44(0) 20 72670159
E-mail: info@dunitz.co.uk
Website: http://www.dunitz.co.uk

Although every effort has been made to ensure that drug doses and other information are presented accurately in this publication, the ultimate responsibility rests with the prescribing physician. Neither the publishers nor the authors can be held responsible for errors or for any consequences arising from the use of information contained herein. For detailed prescribing information or instructions on the use of any product or procedure discussed herein, please consult the prescribing information or instructional material issued by the manufacturer.

A CIP record for this book is available from the British Library.

ISBN 1–901865–87–8

Distributed in the USA by:
Fulfilment Center
Taylor & Francis
7625 Empire Drive
Florence, KY 41042, USA
Toll Free Tel.:   +1 800 634 7064
E-mail: cserve@routledge_ny.com

Distributed in Canada by:
Taylor & Francis
74 Rolark Drive
Scarborough, Ontario M1R 4G2, Canada
Toll Free Tel.:   +1 877 226 2237
E-mail: tal_fran@istar.ca

Distributed in the rest of the world by:
ITPS Limited
Cheriton House
North Way
Andover, Hampshire SP10 5BE, UK
Tel.:   +44 (0)1264 332424
E-mail: reception@itps.co.uk

Composition by J&L Composition Ltd, Filey, North Yorkshire
Printed and bound in Spain by Grafos SA Arte sobre papel

Contents

Preface

Colorectal cancer is one of the major malignancies afflicting westernized societies in terms of both incidence and cause of cancer mortality. In many Western countries, the individual's lifetime risk for this neoplasm is about 5–6%, and approximately half will be long-term survivors.

However, *colorectal cancer is a preventable and treatable disease.* Other than tobacco-related lung cancer, it is the malignancy that has been most extensively studied and understood. Its etiology is complex and multifactorial, including both diet and inherited susceptibility. The pathogenesis of cancer from pre-existing dysplastic lesions, usually adenomas, has been well described. Its relatively easy accessibility to radiologic and endoscopic diagnosis facilitates early detection and even non-surgical therapy by polypectomy. Polypectomy itself will reduce the cancer incidence, while if cancer is detected in the asymptomatic and usually pre-invasive stage, then a surgical cure is possible in almost 90% of the cases.

In spite of this excellent outcome, most westernized countries have not systematically and actively promoted primary and secondary preventive policies for their general population. This is in contrast to the status of breast cancer screening, which has both emotional appeal and, most importantly, political support. Even so, at national levels, we have examples of the health services of Japan, the USA, Israel, and Germany providing a large-bowel screening program *for those who request it.* In addition, nationally budgeted pilot population screening studies have been initiated in the UK and Australia.

However, recently, the national media, key role-model personalities, professional medical societies, medical insurance organizations, individual physicians, and individuals at risk are promoting and demanding preventive medical practices. In the USA, this has led to the inclusion of colorectal cancer screening in the Medicare Program.

In 1996, three of us edited a multi-authored book that brought together the scientific evidence and knowledge relevant to colorectal cancer prevention: Young GP, Rozen P, Levin B (eds), *Prevention and Early Detection of Colorectal Cancer.* London: Saunders. This has been well received by general physicians, as well as specialists, as a reference volume. As new information is being acquired and preventive medicine (including chemoprevention, and changes in diet and lifestyle) is being promoted, we feel that it is important to provide the clinician in practice with an easy to read and up-to-date guide on the primary and secondary prevention of large-bowel neoplasia. This includes primary-care physicians such as family physicians and internists, as well as surgeons, gastroenterologists, oncologists, and public health personnel.

The chapters in this volume provide an up-to-date précis of knowledge and also emphasize the practical preventive steps that can be taken to reduce morbidity and mortality from colorectal cancer (see the Table and Figure). For those who want more information, we have provided recent references and indicated review or general articles on the topics discussed.

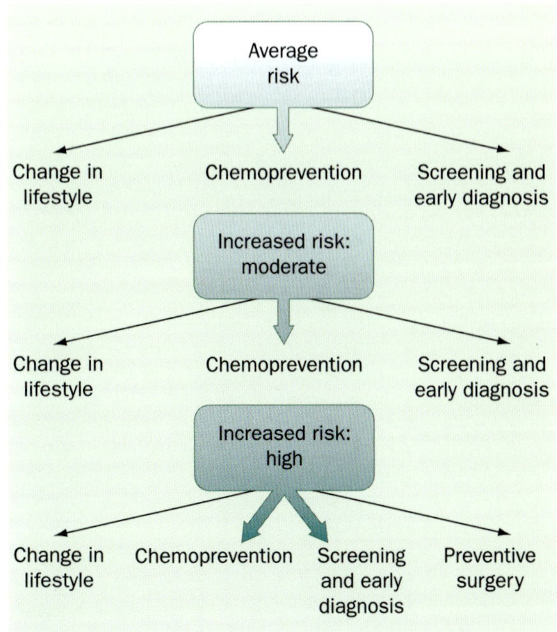

Figure *Algorithm of preventive medical strategies for persons at average or increased risk for colorectal cancer.*

<table>
<tr><td>Table Colorectal cancer: its prevention and management</td></tr>
</table>

- The size of the problem
  - How it might present
- How cancer develops
- Risk factors
  - Diet and chemoprevention
  - Familial risk
  - Premalignant conditions
- Screening
  - Follow-up of high-risk conditions
  - Average-risk screening
- Cancer management
- Public health aspects

We hope that this volume will become a guide for the clinician who has both the first and the on-going contact with the general population, as well as with those at increased risk.

Paul Rozen, Graeme P Young,
Bernard Levin, Stephen J Spann

Acknowledgements

This book is dedicated to our wives, Etta, Joan, Ronnie, and Nancy, for their love, support, and patience. Without the excellent help of our secretaries Sally Zimmerman, Fiona Bertrand, Rosanne Lemon, and Sherry Franovich, it would not have been possible to compile this book – to them we are extremely grateful.

We are also very grateful to Dr John Skibber, Associate Professor, Department of Surgical Oncology, University of Texas MD Anderson Cancer Center, for his contribution to Chapter 9. Finally, we wish to acknowledge our constructive working relationship with the Publishers.

The Authors

Dr Paul Rozen is a gastroenterologist and internist who is a Professor of Medicine at Tel Aviv University and is also at the Department of Gastroenterology, Tel Aviv Medical Center, Tel Aviv. He has received research grants relevant to this publication from Boehringer Mannheim, Germany, SmithKline Diagnostics, and Beckman Coulter, California. His address is: Department of Gastroenterology, Tel Aviv Medical Center, 6 Weizmann St, Tel Aviv 64239, Israel; Fax: +972 3 6974622; E-mail: rozen@tasmc.health.gov.il.

Dr Graeme P Young is a gastroenterologist who is Professor of Gastroenterology at Flinders University of South Australia and the Academic Head of Gastrointestinal Services at Flinders Medical Centre, Adelaide, South Australia. He has been in receipt of research funds from commercial entities relevant to the prevention of bowel cancer: Kelloggs Australia, Uncle Toby's Australia, Starch Australasia, Meadow Lea Corporation Sydney, SmithKline Diagnostics Inc. Sunnyvale, Beckman Coulter Primary Care Diagnostics, Palo Alto, and Enterix Pty Ltd, Sydney. He has also served as a consultant or advisory board member for the following: Starch Australasia, Sanitarium Health Food Corporation Sydney, Enterix Pty Ltd, Boehringer Mannheim, Germany, Encore Pharmaceuticals Los Angeles, and SmithKline Diagnostics Inc. His address is: Department of Gastroenterology and Hepatology, Flinders Medical Centre, Bedford Park (Adelaide), South Australia 5042, Australia; Fax: +61 8 8204 3943; E-mail: graeme.young@flinders.edu.au.

Dr Bernard Levin is a gastroenterologist and internist who is a Professor of Medicine and Vice President of Cancer Prevention at the University of Texas MD Anderson Cancer Center. He has served as a consultant to Searle/Pharmacia in the area of chemoprevention of colorectal neoplasia. His address is: Bernard Levin, MD, Division of Cancer Prevention, University of Texas MD Anderson Cancer Center, 1515 Holcombe Boulevard, Box 203, Houston, TX 77030, USA; Fax: +1713 792 0629; E-mail: blevin@mdanderson.org.

Dr Stephen J Spann is a family physician who is Professor and the Richard M Kleberg, Sr Chair of the Department of Family and Community Medicine at Baylor College of Medicine. His address is: Stephen J Spann, MD, Department of Family and Community Medicine, Baylor College of Medicine, 5510 Greenbriar, Houston, TX 77005, USA; Fax: +1713 798 7778; E-mail: sspann@bcm.tmc.edu.

Colorectal cancer: How big is the problem, why prevent it, and how might it present?

Stephen J Spann, Paul Rozen, Bernard Levin, Graeme P Young

The size of the problem

Colorectal cancer is one of the most commonly diagnosed cancers, and a leading cause of cancer deaths, around the world. The high incidence countries include all of North America, Western Europe, Japan, Australia, and New Zealand. They also include Argentina, Israel, Singapore, Hong Kong, and parts of Malaysia. The relative incidence of different cancers varies with a country's level of economic development. In the developed regions of the world, colorectal cancer is the third most common malignancy after lung and stomach in males and after breast in women (Tables 1.1 and 1.2; see also Chapter 2, Figures 2.1 and 2.4). However, in terms of national health burden, mortality reflects not only incidence, but also availability of diagnostic services and therapy. As can be seen in Figure 1.1, mortality from colorectal cancer is very high throughout Eastern Europe and what was previously known as the Soviet Union, as well as in most of the other countries mentioned above. In 1990, it was the fourth most common cancer diagnosed and the fourth most common cause of cancer mortality in men worldwide; and the third most common cancer diagnosed and the fourth

most common cause of cancer mortality in women.[1] In the USA, for example, colorectal cancer is the third most commonly diagnosed cancer, with an estimated 130 200 new cases in the year 2000; it is the second leading cause of cancer mortality there, accounting for an estimated 56 300 deaths in that year.[2] The cost of treating patients with colorectal cancer is significant. It is estimated that in the USA, these costs approach $6.5 billion per year. This is second in cancer treatment costs only to breast cancer, at $6.6 billion per year, and exceeds the costs of treating lung cancer at $5.1 billion per year and prostate cancer at $4.7 billion per year.[3]

Time trends

In some developed countries, both the incidence and mortality rates for colorectal cancer have been stable or even declining[4] (Figures 1.2 and 1.3). Declining incidence rates may reflect a change in lifestyle, earlier detection, and treatment of polyps before these advance to carcinomas. Declining mortality rates are felt to reflect both the decreasing incidence of disease, along with earlier detection in some individuals. In the US population, the greatest reduction in incidence and mortality has occurred in White

Table 1.1 *Age-standardized rates of cancer incidence (per 100 000) for males by site: select regions, 1990[a]*

	Esophagus	Stomach	COLON/RECTUM	Liver	Lung	Prostate
Northern Africa	2.8	5.9	**6.0**	4.7	12.8	5.1
Western Africa	2.1	12.4	**4.7**	22.1	2.2	23.9
Central America	3.4	18.6	**8.8**	5.4	19.3	24.8
South America (tropical)	7.7	31.1	**15.0**	3.2	24.1	28.1
North America	5.2	8.4	**44.3**	3.2	69.6	92.4
Eastern Asia: China	21.6	43.6	**13.3**	35.8	34.7	1.1
Eastern Asia: Japan	9.5	77.9	**39.5**	27.6	38.9	8.5
South central Asia	9.0	6.7	**5.0**	2.8	11.9	4.5
Western Europe	6.9	16.4	**39.8**	4.9	54.1	39.6
Australia/New Zealand	4.6	10.8	**45.8**	2.8	47.6	49.7

[a] Adapted from reference 1.

Table 1.2 Age-standardized rates of cancer incidence (per 100 000) for females by site: select regions, 1990[a]

	Esophagus	Stomach	COLON/ RECTUM	Liver	Lung	Breast	Cervix
Northern Africa	1.7	2.6	**4.2**	2.4	2.6	25.0	11.3
Western Africa	1.2	6.6	**3.9**	6.7	0.9	19.0	26.2
Central America	1.4	13.3	**7.9**	4.0	7.9	25.5	44.4
South America (tropical)	2.0	15.9	**13.6**	2.2	7.2	39.1	31.8
North America	1.4	4.0	**32.8**	1.4	32.9	86.3	9.1
Eastern Asia: China	9.9	19.0	**10.2**	11.5	13.4	11.8	5.0
Eastern Asia: Japan	1.6	33.3	**24.6**	6.9	11.2	28.6	9.7
South central Asia	7.0	4.0	**3.8**	1.5	2.6	21.2	23.8
Western Europe	1.1	8.2	**29.0**	1.5	8.2	67.3	10.9
Australia/New Zealand	2.4	4.9	**34.8**	1.1	16.1	71.7	11.2

[a] Adapted from reference 1.

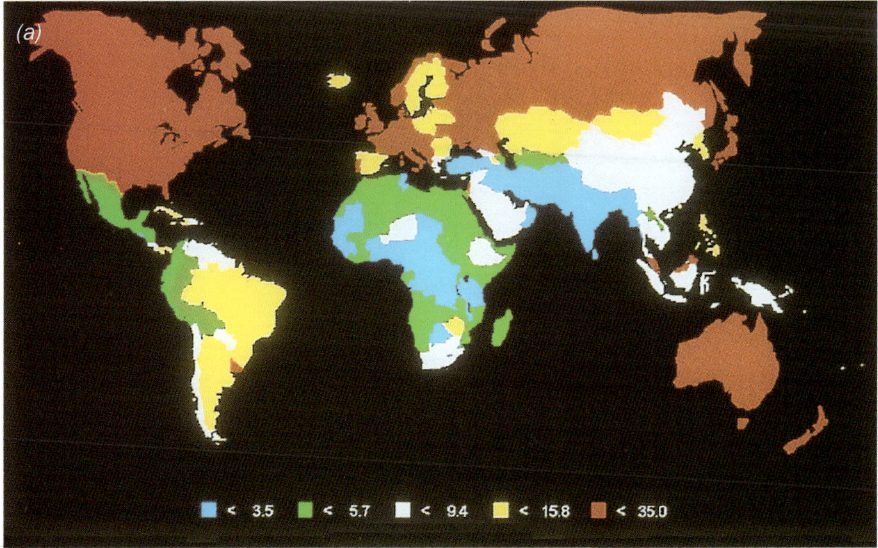

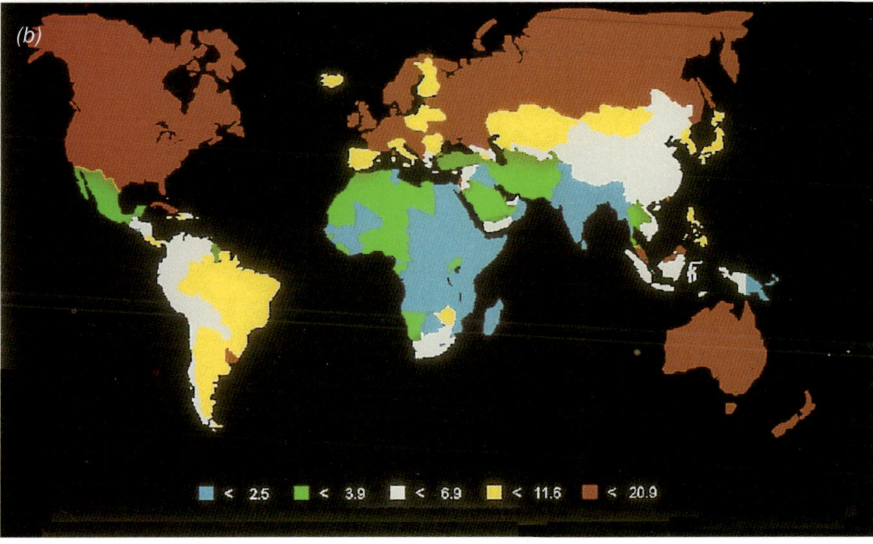

Figure 1.1 Worldwide range of colorectal cancer mortality in countries having a 'westernized' lifestyle (age-standardized mortality rate): (a) males; (b) females. Prepared by Dr A Zauber and derived from reference 1.

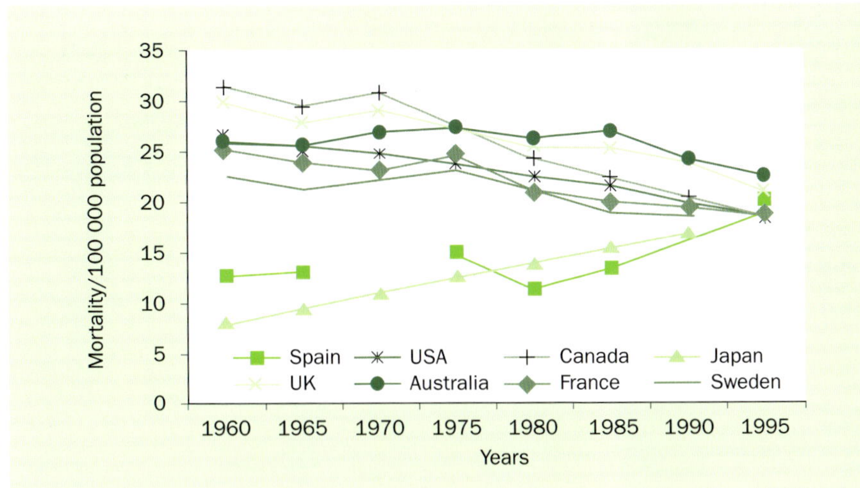

Figure 1.2 *Mortality from colorectal cancer in different countries worldwide. In some, mortality is increasing, while in others, it has remained with little change. Based on data derived from reference 4.*

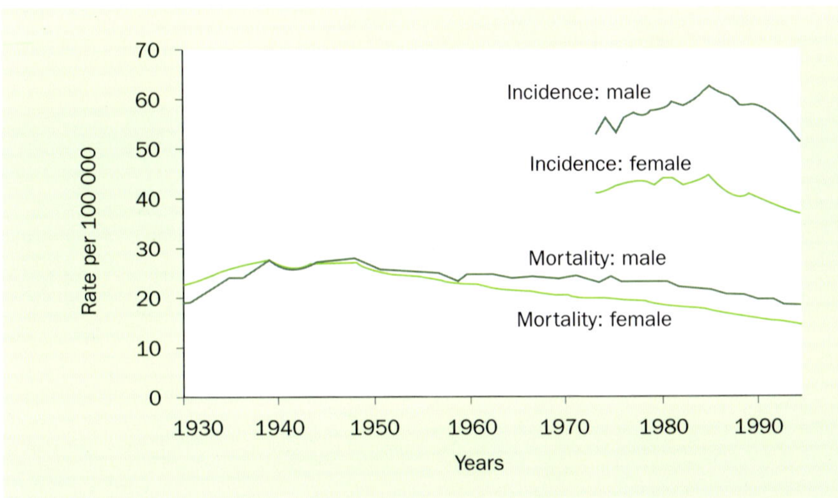

Figure 1.3 *Colorectal cancer incidence (1973–1995) and mortality (1930–1995) in the US population. There has been a recent fall in incidence in both sexes, and a reduction in mortality in females, especially in White women. Reprinted by permission of the American Cancer Society Inc.*

women (Figures 1.3 and 1.4). But, in the corresponding period, there was actually an increased mortality in African-American men of 21% and women of 7%.[2]

In other countries that have an improving socio-economic level and a 'westernized' lifestyle, there has been a parallel rising incidence of large-bowel neoplasia (Figure 1.4).[9] These include countries from regions as diverse as Eastern Europe, Asia, and Latin America.

Risk factors for colorectal cancer

A number of factors appear to increase an individual's risk for colorectal cancer, including older age, male gender, diet and exercise habits, a personal history of inflammatory bowel disease, certain genetic syndromes, and a family history of colorectal cancer or adenomatous polyps (see Chapters 2, 4, and 6). Adenomatous polyps are the precursors of most colorectal cancers; removal of these polyps appears to lower the incidence of subsequent colorectal cancer.[10]

Stage at diagnosis and mortality

Colorectal cancer survival is closely related to the clinical and pathologic stage of the disease at diagnosis. The commonly used classifications of staging are given in Table 1.3. The 5-year survival rate is approximately 90% in patients with cancers limited to the bowel wall, compared with 60% of those with lymph node involvement, and less than 10% of patients with metastatic disease at the time

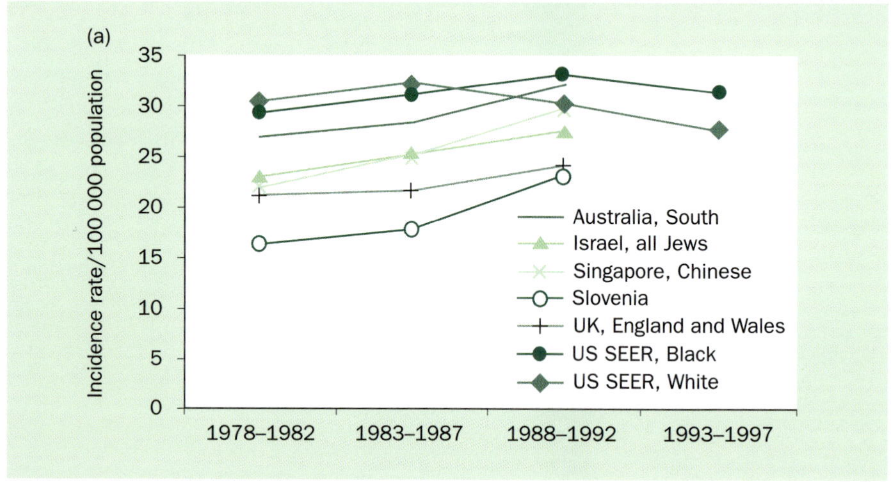
(a)
35
30
25
20
15
10
5
0
Incidence rate/100 000 population
Australia, South
Israel, all Jews
Singapore, Chinese
Slovenia
UK, England and Wales
US SEER, Black
US SEER, White
1978–1982
1983–1987
1988–1992
1993–1997

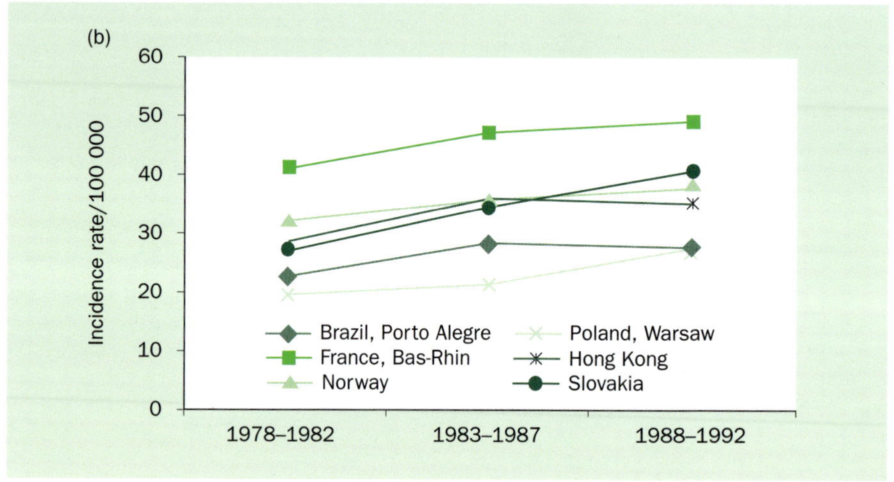
(b)
60
50
40
30
20
10
0
Incidence rate/100 000
Brazil, Porto Alegre
France, Bas-Rhin
Norway
Poland, Warsaw
Hong Kong
Slovakia
1978–1982
1983–1987
1988–1992

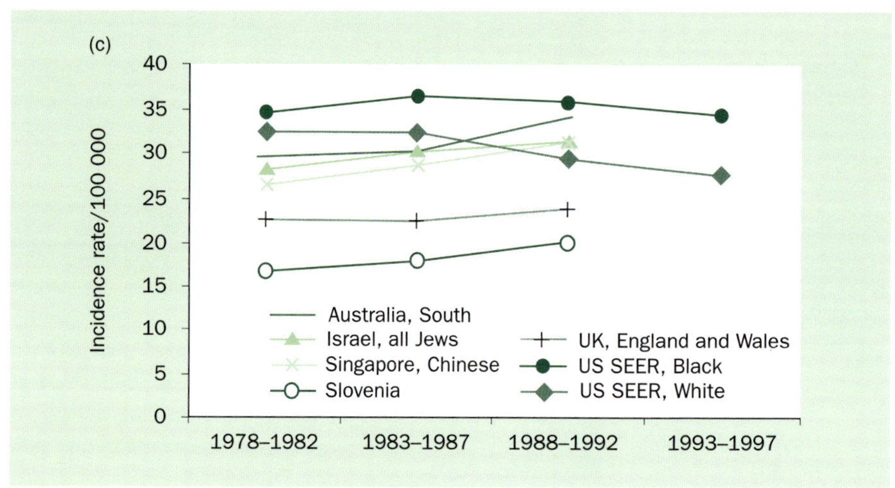
(c)
40
35
30
25
20
15
10
5
0
Incidence rate/100 000
Australia, South
Israel, all Jews
Singapore, Chinese
Slovenia
UK, England and Wales
US SEER, Black
US SEER, White
1978–1982
1983–1987
1988–1992
1993–1997

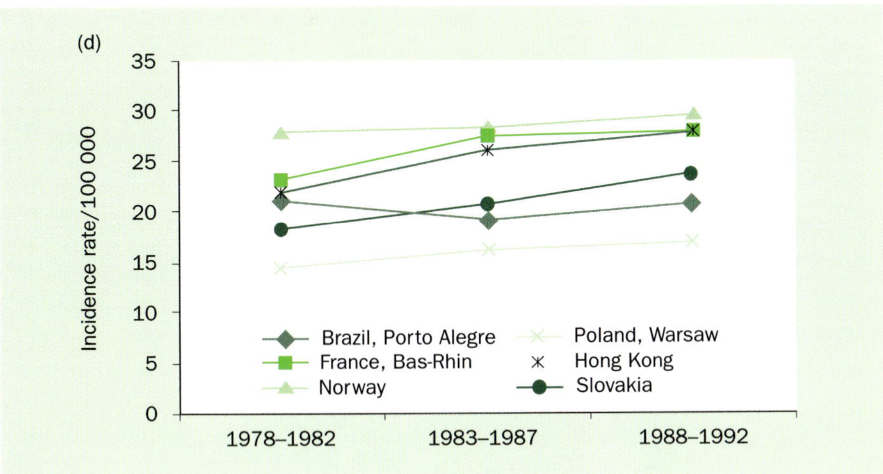

Figure 1.4 *Changes with time in incidence of colorectal cancer in diverse developed countries and those in transition: (a,b) male; (c,d) female. Data shown, including the US SEER data,[5] are age-standardized as used in references 6–8. Note the high but falling incidence in the US White, as compared with the Black population and the rising incidence worldwide in males in diverse westernized countries.*

of diagnosis[11] (Table 1.3). This emphasizes the fact that if colorectal cancer is detected at an early, asymptomatic stage, then we should expect decreased morbidity and mortality from the disease (secondary prevention) (see Chapter 8).

Screening for cancer

Secondary prevention offered to an entire population at average risk for a given disease is called 'screening' for that disease. When secondary prevention is targeted at individuals who have one or more risk factors for a given disease, it is called 'case-finding'. A number of expert panels have suggested the application of specific criteria for deciding whether or not a given disease is amenable to secondary prevention.[12,13] The criteria required by the US Preventive Services Task Force include the following:

- The target condition (disease being screened for) must cause a significant burden of suffering: it must be relatively common, in terms of prevalence and incidence, and it must be clinically significant in terms of morbidity and mortality
- The screening test must be able to detect the target condition earlier than without screening, and with sufficient accuracy to avoid producing large numbers of false-positive and false-negative results
- Screening for and treating persons with early disease should improve the likelihood of favorable health outcomes, such as decreased disease-specific morbidity or mortality, compared with treating patients when they present with symptoms and signs of the disease.[12]

False-negative test results can lead to false reassurance and a missed opportunity for early detection and treatment of the disease. *False-positive test* results usually lead to additional diagnostic tests and their associated expense and potential risk, as well as to psychological anxiety in the patient who thinks he or she might have the disease. Test *sensitivity* is the probability that the test will be abnormal in a patient who has the disease

Table 1.3 *Relationship between 5-year survival rate and stage at diagnosis[a]*

Stage at diagnosis			
	Dukes (modified)	**TNM**	**5-year survival rate (%)**
Limited to bowel wall	A and B	Stage 1	90
Regional node involvement	C	Stages 2 and 3	60
Distant metastases	D	Stage 4	10

[a] Adapted from reference 11.

of interest. The higher the sensitivity of a test, the lower its false-negative rate. Test *specificity* is the probability that the test will be normal in a patient who does not have the disease of interest. The higher the specificity of a test, the lower its false-positive rate. See Table 1.4.

Clinicians are also interested in the predictive values of test results (Table 1.4). *Positive predictive value* is the probability that a patient with a positive test does, in fact, have the disease of interest. *Negative predictive* value is the probability that a patient with a negative test is, in fact, free of the disease of interest. Positive predictive value is directly proportional to test specificity: the higher the specificity of a test, the higher its positive predictive value. Negative predictive value is directly proportional to test sensitivity; the higher the sensitivity of a test, the higher its negative predictive value. Positive predictive value is directly proportional to the prevalence of the disease in the population tested: when screening a population at average risk for a given cancer, the positive predictive value will be low, since the prevalence rate will be low, by definition. Negative predictive value is indirectly proportional to the prevalence of disease in the population tested: in the average-risk screening situation, the negative predictive value will be high. In other words, most positive screening tests will be falsely positive, and the overwhelming majority of negative screening tests will be truly negative.

Table 1.4 Definitions of terms describing screening tests and their interpretation

Term	Definition
True-negative	Non-diseased patient has a negative (normal) test
True-positive	Diseased patient has a positive (abnormal) test
False-negative	Diseased patient has a negative (normal) test
False-positive	Non-diseased patient has a positive (abnormal) test
Sensitivity (true-positive rate)	Probability that a diseased patient will have a positive (abnormal) test
Specificity (true-negative rate)	Probability that a non-diseased patient will have a negative (normal) test
Positive predictive value	Probability that a patient with a positive (abnormal) test does have the disease
Negative predictive value	Probability that a patient with a negative (normal) test does not have the disease

It can be challenging to establish that a screening test really leads to improved health outcomes; this is especially true for cancer screening tests. For most types of cancer, 5–year survival is higher for individuals identified with early-stage disease. It is tempting to conclude that early detection is effective because death appears to be delayed as a result of screening and early treatment. However, survival data may be influenced by *lead-time* bias: survival may appear to be lengthened when in fact screening has only advanced the time of diagnosis, lengthening the period of time between diagnosis and death without any true prolongation of life (Figure 1.5). Length bias can also cause unduly optimistic estimates of the effectiveness of screening for cancer: screening tests have a tendency to detect slowly growing tumors, since fast growing tumors become symptomatic quicker. Patients found by screening may do better than unscreened patients even if the screening itself doesn't really affect the outcome. To determine whether or not a cancer-screening test is truly efficacious, it is best to conduct a randomized clinical trial, in which the experimental group receives the screening intervention of interest, and the control group does not. Both groups are then followed over time, and disease-specific mortality for that cancer is compared between the two groups. A randomized clinical trial showing decreased disease-specific mortality in the screening intervention group provides the most robust evidence of screening efficacy.[12,13]

The best example of an accepted and promoted cancer-screening program is that of using mammography for breast cancer. This is actively promoted in many Western countries and has become the 'gold standard' when evaluating cost-effectiveness of other proposed cancer-screening programs such as prostate or colorectal neoplasia screening.

Screening studies for colorectal cancer
Fecal occult blood testing

Fecal occult blood testing (FOBT) as a screening test for colorectal cancer meets these criteria. Three randomized trials have shown that FOBT is both efficacious and effective in lowering colorectal cancer mortality in individuals who undergo screening.

Mandel and colleagues[14] studied 46 551 participants 50–80 years of age from the US state of Minnesota who agreed to be randomized to annual, biennial, or no screening for colorectal cancer with FOBT, using six guaiac-impregnated paper slides with two smears from each of three consecutive stools. Eighty-three percent of slides were rehydrated. Participants with a positive test were evaluated with colonoscopy. The 13-year cumulative

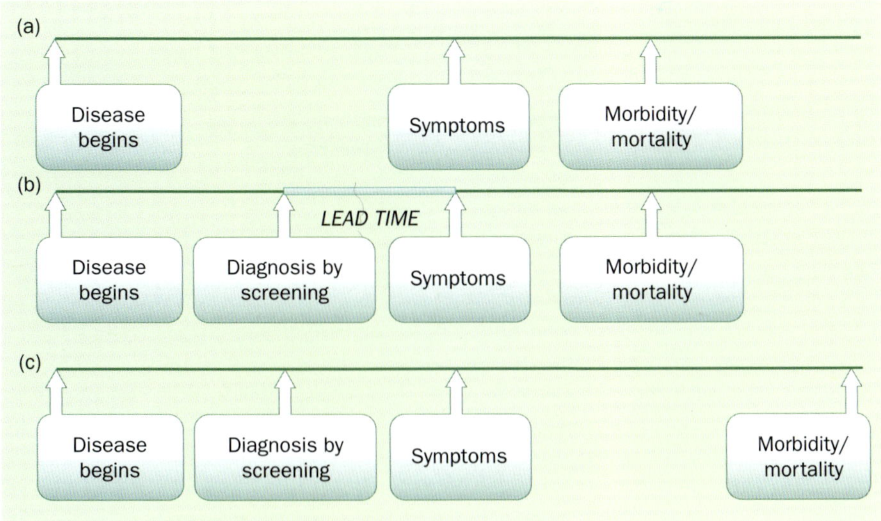

Figure 1.5 *Line (a) depicts the natural history of disease in the absence of a screening test. Line (b) depicts lead-time bias: although the diagnosis of disease is made earlier with the screening test because of the lead time, the ultimate outcome of disease (morbidity/mortality) has not changed. Line (c) depicts the benefits of a good screening test: early detection, in time through screening, changes the outcome by preventing or postponing morbidity/mortality.*

mortality per 1000 from colorectal cancer was 5.88 in the annually screened group, 8.33 in the biennially screened group, and 8.83 in the control group. Annual FOBT screening reduced the 13-year cumulative colorectal mortality by 33%. The number needed to screen annually to prevent one death from colorectal cancer during the 13-year follow-up period was 339 individuals.

Kronborg and colleagues[15] randomized a population of 137 485 people aged 45–75 living in Funen, Denmark to an invitation to biennial FOBT screening during a 10-year period (30 967), no invitation to screening (30 966), or non-enrollment in the study (75 552). During the 10-year study, 481 people in the screening group had a diagnosis of colorectal cancer, compared with 483 in the unscreened control group. There were only 205 deaths attributable to colorectal cancer in the screened group, compared with 249 deaths in the control group, with a significant reduction in mortality of 18%. The number needed to screen biennially to prevent one death from colorectal cancer during the 10-year study period was 704 individuals.

Hardcastle and colleagues,[16] over a 10-year period, randomized a population of 152 850 individuals 45–74 years of age living in the Nottingham area of the UK to biennial FOBT screening (76 466) or control (76 384). The median follow-up was 7.8 years. In the screening group, 360 individuals died from colorectal cancer compared with 420 in the control group, with a significant 15% reduction in cumulative colorectal cancer mortality in the screened group. The number needed to screen biennially to prevent one death from colorectal cancer during the follow-up period in this study was 1275 individuals.

The different effect sizes in these studies undoubtedly relate to the different screening methods used: unhydrated or rehydrated FOBT, test intervals and different lengths of follow-up (Table 1.5). The Minnesota study, with the greatest effect size (and smallest number needed to screen), had the shortest screening interval and the longest follow-up period. The Nottingham study, with the smallest effect size (and largest number needed to screen), had the longest screening interval, and the shortest median follow-up period.

Screening sigmoidoscopy

The data on screening sigmoidoscopy are not quite as robust; there are no results available from randomized trials of this procedure. However, three case–control studies provide evidence that screening sigmoidoscopy can reduce mortality from colorectal cancer. Selby and colleagues[17] compared the screening history of individuals who died from colorectal cancer with that of matched controls. Rigid sigmoidoscopy was associated with a 59% reduction in risk of death from colorectal cancer located in a part of the colon reachable by the sigmoidoscope. Newcomb and colleagues[18] found an 80% reduction in the risk of death from rectosigmoid cancer in patients who had undergone one or more sigmoidoscopies, compared with

Table 1.5 Summary of randomized controlled trials of screening for colon cancer with fecal occult blood testing (FOBT): their performance and efficacy

Study	FOBT rehydration	Screening interval	Years of follow-up	Percentage reduction in colorectal cancer mortality	No. needed to screen/cancer diagnosed
Mandel et al[14]	Yes	Annual	13	33	339
Kronborg et al[15]	No	Biennial	10	18	704
Hardcastle et al[16]	No	Biennial	7.8	15	1275

those who had never done so. Muller and Sonnenberg[19] evaluated 4411 US veterans who died of colorectal cancer and matched controls, finding that proctosigmoidoscopy reduced mortality from colorectal cancer in the area examined by approximately 60%. These studies suggest that sigmoidoscopy is efficacious in reducing colorectal cancer mortality risk.

The combination of FOBT and sigmoidoscopy, compared with sigmoidoscopy alone as a colorectal cancer-screening strategy, was evaluated in one controlled trial. Patients were assigned to one or the other screening intervention according to the date of screening. Colorectal cancer mortality was lower in the group receiving the combined screening procedure.[20]

Randomized population trials of sigmoidoscopy, with or without FOBT, are taking place in the US, UK, and Norway. No data are available yet on colorectal cancer mortality.[21]

The above trials and studies have provided the evidence for the recommendations in the Colorectal Screening Guidelines of the World Health Organization (WHO) Colorectal Cancer Collaborative Group, the US Preventive Services Task Force, the American Cancer Society, and the American Gastroenterological Association.[22–24] These have been adopted by Medicare (the universal health insurance provided to US citizens from the age of 65 years)[25] (Table 1.6). Similar screening programs, or variations, have been initiated or are in place in other countries such as Japan, Australia, and Israel.[21]

Screening colonoscopy

There are no results available from randomized studies of screening colonoscopy to demonstrate a significant reduction in colorectal mortality in the average-risk population. Nor has it been shown to be more effective and/or less costly than the previously described methods. Such studies are in progress. Even so, the clinical evidence supporting screening colonoscopy is strong.[24] This has led to its inclusion by Medicare as an alternative screening method,

Table 1.6 Colorectal cancer screening tests covered by the US Medicare insurance plan[a]

Patient risk status	Fecal occult blood test	Flexible sigmoidoscopy	Colonoscopy	Barium enema
Average risk (age = 50 years)	Once every 12 months	Once every 48 months	Once every 10 years	May substitute for flexible sigmoidoscopy if physician determines that it will be equally effective for that individual
High risk (positive family history, previous colorectal cancer or precursor neoplastic polyps, history of inflammatory bowel disease, presence of appropriate gene markers, or other predisposing factors)			Once every 24 months	May substitute for colonoscopy if physician determines that it will be equally effective for that individual

[a] Adapted from reference 25.

once in 10 years. The Italian National Health Authorities have also made 5-yearly screening colonoscopy available for the average-risk population (personal communication, Dr M Crespi, Rome).

Compliance

Despite the proven efficacy of these screening tests for colorectal cancer, most individuals living in countries in which they are routinely recommended and offered do not participate in screening. In the USA, data from the National Health Interview Survey showed that in 1992 only 17.3% of individuals 50 years of age or older had FOBT performed in the previous year, and only 9.4% had undergone sigmoidoscopy during the previous 3 years.[26,27] An analysis of the 1992 and 1993 Behavior Risk Surveillance System conducted by the Centers for Disease Control and Prevention documented low use of colorectal cancer screening tests in the USA, and underscored the need for efforts to increase screening.[28] Lieberman[29] has estimated that a 50% population compliance rate with an FOBT screening program would result in a 24% reduction in mortality from colorectal cancer, equivalent to 13 512 deaths prevented in the USA for the year 2000. The issues of compliance for screening tests are addressed in Chapter 10.

Symptoms and signs of colorectal cancer

Ideally, the majority of patients with colorectal cancer would be identified through screening, in an early, asymptomatic stage, with a high probability of cure. Regrettably, many patients today are still diagnosed because of symptoms of established disease, and only 10–15% of these patients are found to have an early-stage cancer.[15,30] Nonetheless, clinicians must remain alert for symptoms and signs that suggest the possibility of colorectal cancer, and be prepared to conduct the appropriate evaluation to rule out this disease.

Clinical presentation and evaluation

The clinical presentation of large-bowel cancer is dependent on its location within the colon and rectum, as well as the extent of spread. Right-sided lesions may present with abdominal pain, weakness (due to anemia), melena, and an abdominal mass. Left-sided lesions may also present with abdominal pain and melena, or bright red rectal bleeding, but constipation is also fairly common. Rectosigmoid and rectal lesions often present with bright red rectal bleeding, constipation, and tenesmus. Narrowing of the stool diameter is also common. The absence of con-stipation in the presence of right-sided lesions is due to the presence of liquid contents in the right side of the colon and the larger luminal capacity compared with the narrower lumen of the rectosigmoid and rectum.

The work-up of a patient with a suspected colorectal cancer includes a complete history, physical examination, and selected laboratory and radiologic tests. The history includes the patient's symptoms, prior removal of an adenoma or cancer, previous inflammatory bowel disease, and a family history of colorectal neoplasia or one of the inherited colorectal cancer syndromes. Physical examination may reveal evidence of Peutz–Jeghers or Gardner's syndrome or may suggest spread to the liver, peritoneal cavity, or lymph nodes. A digital rectal examination is necessary to determine the presence of a distal rectal cancer or of pelvic spread. In women, a thorough pelvic examination is required.

Laboratory tests may reveal liver enzyme abnormalities or iron deficiency anemia. In selected patients, a CEA (carcinoembryonic antigen) determination may be appropriate (see the discussion of postoperative surveillance in Chapter 9).

Colonoscopy is the preferred approach for evaluating the patient with suspected large-bowel cancer. Another approach is to use flexible sigmoidoscopy followed by double-contrast barium enema. Colonoscopy is also indicated for examining patients in whom an abnormality has been detected on barium enema; in addition, the presence of synchronous cancers and adenomas can be determined.

Computed tomography (CT) of the abdomen and pelvis may aid in determining the extent of spread. A chest radiograph will help to evaluate the possibility of lung metastasis. Endoscopic ultrasonography is being used more frequently to help in the staging of rectal cancers, and depth of invasion can often be determined with accuracy.

The predictive value of common symptoms and signs

The frequency of presenting symptoms and signs varies by study and by location of the tumor in the bowel[31–33] (Tables 1.7 and 1.8). Of course, not all patients who present with these types of symptoms and signs have colorectal cancer: their positive predictive value for this disease is only moderate, and depends on the patient population. Studies evaluating patients with symptomatic rectal bleeding in general practice have shown positive predictive values for colon cancer ranging between 3.3% and 15.5%, and positive predictive values for adenomatous polyps ranging between 2.2% and 25%[34–36] (Table 1.9).

Table 1.7 *Frequency (%) of presenting symptoms and signs in patients diagnosed with colorectal cancer in different published series*

Study	Rectal bleeding	Abdominal pain	Change in bowel habits	Anemia	Positive FOBT
Majumdar et al[31]	58	52	51	57	77
Kyle et al[32]	44	41	56		
Speights et al[30]	34	22			

Table 1.8 *Frequency (%) of presenting symptoms and signs of colorectal cancer, according to tumor location, in different series*

Study	Tumor location	Abdominal pain	Rectal bleeding	Fatigue/ weakness	Weight loss	Change in bowel habits	Abnormal stools	Anemia	Abdominal mass	Abdominal tenderness	Rectal mass	Obstruction
Majumdar et al[31]	Proximal		73	31	46			70				
	Distal		70		34	30	30	47				
Lanier et al[33]	Proximal	62		38		30			37	28	23	
	Distal	42	68			68				12	61	18

Table 1.9 *The predictive value of rectal bleeding in the general practice setting*

Study	Study location	No. of patients	Patient ages (years)	Percentage with cancer	Percentage with polyps
Fijten et al[34]	Netherlands	269	18–75	3.3	2.2
Metcalf et al[35]	UK	99	>40	8	25
Norrelund and Norrelund[36]	Denmark	208	≥40	15.5	7.7
Norrelund and Norrelund[36]	Denmark	156	≥40	14.1	11.5

Rex[37] reviewed the literature on the diagnostic yield of colonoscopies performed on patients with various findings and symptoms suggestive of colorectal cancer. In 12 studies with a combined 1655 patients, reporting on colonoscopy results in patients with non-emergent rectal bleeding, the average prevalence of colorectal cancer was 11% (range 4–29%), and the average prevalence of adenomatous polyps was 22% (range 13–42%). In four studies with a combined 641 patients reporting on colonoscopy results in patients with symptoms of abdominal pain and/or change in bowel habits without rectal bleeding, the average prevalence of colon cancer was 2.8% (range 0–5%), and the average risk of adenomatous polyps was 16% (range 6–31%). Neugut and colleagues[38] evaluated the diagnostic yield of colonoscopy for patients with abdominal pain, change in bowel habits, and rectal bleeding, referred to three colonoscopy practices in New York City between 1986 and 1989. Patients with rectal bleeding were again found to have a higher prevalence of colorectal cancer and adenomatous polyps than patients with other presenting symptoms (Table 1.10). Thus, it would appear that rectal bleeding is a more ominous symptom than are abdominal pain and/or change in bowel habits without rectal bleeding.

What is the appropriate work-up of a symptomatic patient?

There are two methods of imaging the entire colon: colonoscopy, and flexible sigmoidoscopy plus double-contrast barium enema. Colonoscopy is better for the

Table 1.10 *Diagnostic outcomes of colonscopies performed on referred patients with common symptoms of colorectal cancer*[a]

Symptom	No. of patients	Percentage with colorectal cancer	Percentage with adenomatous polyps
Rectal bleeding	861	8.6	25
Abdominal pain	113	4.4	17.7
Change in bowel habits	154	5.8	21.4
Abdominal pain and change in bowel habits	44	6.8	15.9

[a] Adapted from reference 38.

detection of small adenomas, and provides an opportunity for biopsy and polypectomy. Flexible sigmoidoscopy plus double-contrast barium enema has a sensitivity comparable to colonoscopy for detection of cancers and large polyps, and may be less expensive than colonoscopy in some settings. Irvine and colleagues[39] compared double-contrast barium enema plus flexible sigmoidoscopy versus colonoscopy in the evaluation of 71 patients with overt rectal bleeding. Patients were evaluated with all tests, and the results of the combination of tests was used as the gold standard. Colonoscopy was found to be 82% sensitive for diagnosing adenoma or carcinoma, compared with a sensitivity of 73% for double-contrast barium enema plus flexible sigmoidoscopy. The positive predictive value of colonoscopy was 87%, compared with 91% for barium enema plus sigmoidoscopy. Jensen and colleagues[40] reported on the diagnostic accuracy of combined double-contrast barium enema plus rectosigmoidoscopy in the evaluation of 530 FOBT-positive patients identified through a randomized trial of colorectal cancer screening of individuals aged 60–64 living in Göteborg, Sweden. Patients with negative work-ups had repeat FOBT, and positives underwent colonoscopy. Patients were followed longitudinally using local cancer and death registries. The combined test strategy was found to have a sensitivity of 90% for colorectal cancers, and a sensitivity of 96% for adenomas at least 1 cm in diameter. Rex and colleagues[41] randomized 380 patients with non-emergent

rectal bleeding, aged 40 years and over, to evaluation with flexible sigmoidoscopy plus air-contrast barium enema versus colonoscopy. Initial colonoscopy detected more polyps less than 9 mm in size, adenomas, and arteriovenous malformations, but fewer cases of diverticulosis. No significant difference was found between strategies in the number of patients found with cancers or polyps greater than 9 mm. Cancers were more common in subjects aged 55 years or more (8%) than in those younger than 55 years (1%). The authors conclude that flexible sigmoidoscopy plus air-contrast barium enema may be more cost-effective in evaluating patients with rectal bleeding younger than 55 years, but colonoscopy may be the more cost-effective strategy in older patients. In a subsequent study of similar design involving 156 patients with colorectal cancer symptoms without rectal bleeding, Rex and colleagues[42] found more adenomas in the initial colonoscopy group, but more diverticulosis in the sigmoidoscopy plus barium enema group. The overall prevalence of cancer (0.6%) and significant adenomas (4.6%) was low. The authors suggest that for this group of patients with symptoms other than rectal bleeding, sigmoidoscopy plus barium enema may be the more cost-effective evaluation strategy, especially for individuals under 55 years of age.

While colonoscopy is clearly the most sensitive test for evaluating patients with symptoms and signs suggestive of colorectal cancer, it may not always be readily available, or affordable. When this is the case, flexible sigmoidoscopy plus double-contrast barium enema may be an acceptable alternative diagnostic strategy. Because this testing strategy is less sensitive, every effort should be made to obtain a colonoscopy in symptomatic patients at highest risk of colorectal cancer: individuals 50 years of age and older who present with rectal bleeding or anemia.

Conclusions

Colorectal cancer constitutes an important cause of morbidity and mortality worldwide. Efficacious and effective screening tests are available that improve disease outcomes. And yet, current compliance with screening recommendations in suboptimal, and needs to be improved. Clinicians must remain alert for symptoms and signs of established disease, as well. Patients displaying such findings should undergo complete visualization of the large intestine, preferably by colonoscopy.

References (*Reviews and general articles)

1. *Ferlay J, Parkin DM, Pisani P, Globocan 1. Cancer incidence and mortality worldwide in 1990. International Agency for Research on Cancer, World Health Organization, http://www-dep.iarc.fr/dataava/globocan/globoJava.html.

2. http://www.cancer.org/statistics/cff2000/selectedcancers.html.

3. *Schrag D, Weeks J, Costs and cost-effectiveness of colorectal cancer prevention and therapy. *Semin Oncol* 1999; **26:** 561–8.

4. Organization for Economic Cooperation and Development, OECD Health Data 99, A Comparative Analysis of 29 Countries. CD ROM published by the Organization for Economic Cooperation and Development.

5. Ries LAG, Eisner MP, Kosary CL et al (eds), *SEER Cancer Statistics Review, 1973–1997*. Bethesda, MD: National Cancer Institute, 2000. *http://seer.cancer.gov/Publications/CSR1973_1997/*.

6. Muir C, Waterhouse J, Mack T et al (eds), *Cancer Incidence in Five Continents,* Vol V. Lyon: IARC Scientific Publication 88, 1987.

7. Parkin DM, Muir CS, Whelan SL et al (eds), *Cancer Incidence in Five Continents*, Vol VI. Lyon: IARC Scientific Publication 120, 1992.

8. Parkin DM, Whelan SL, Ferlay J et al (eds), *Cancer Incidence in Five Continents*. Vol VII. Lyon: IARC Scientific Publication 143, 1997.

9. Bonithon-Kopp C, Benhamiche AM, Are there several colorectal cancers? Epidemiological data. *Eur J Cancer Prev* 1999; **8:** S3–12.

10. *Winawer SJ, Zauber AG, Ho MN et al, Prevention of colorectal cancer by colonoscopic polypectomy. The National Polyp Study Workgroup. *N Engl J Med* 1993; **329:** 1977–81.

11. Greenlee RT, Murray T, Bolden S et al, Cancer statistics, 2000. *CA Cancer J Clin* 2000; **50:** 7–33.

12. *US Preventive Services Task Force, Screening for colorectal cancer. In: *Guide to Clinical Preventive Services*. Baltimore: Williams & Wilkins, 1996: 89–103.

13. The Canadian Task Force on the Periodic Health Examination, Screening for colorectal cancer. In: *The Canadian Guide to Clinical Preventive Health Care. (*Solomon M, McLeod R, eds). Ottawa: Canada Communication Group–Publishing, 1994: 797–807.

14. *Mandel JS, Bond JH, Church TR et al, Reducing mortality from colorectal cancer by screening for fecal occult blood. *N Engl J Med* 1993; **328:** 1365–71.

15. Kronborg O, Fenger C, Olsen J et al, Randomised study of screening for colorectal cancer with faecal-occult-blood test. *Lancet* 1996; **348:** 1467–71.

16. Hardcastle JD, Chamberlain JO, Robinson MHE et al, Randomised controlled trial of faecal-occult-blood screening for colorectal cancer. *Lancet* 1996; **348:** 1472–77.

17. Selby JV, Friedman GD, Quesenberry CP Jr et al, A case–control study of screening sigmoidoscopy and mortality from colorectal cancer. *N Engl J Med* 1992; **326:** 653–7.

18. Newcomb PA, Norfleet RG, Storer BE et al, Screening sigmoidoscopy and colorectal cancer mortality. *J Natl Cancer Inst* 1992; **84:** 1572–5.

19. Muller AD, Sonnenberg A, Prevention of colorectal cancer by flexible endoscopy and polypectomy. A case–control study of 32,702 veterans. *Ann Intern Med* 1995; **123:** 904–10.

20. Winawer SJ, Flehinger BJ, Schottenfeld D et al, Screening for colorectal cancer with fecal occult blood testing and sigmoidoscopy. *J Natl Cancer Inst* 1993; **85:** 1311–18.

21. *Rozen P, The OMED Colorectal Cancer Screening Committee: a report of its aims and activities. *Gastrointest Endosc* 1999; **50:** 449–54.

22. Winawer SJ, St John DJ, Bond JH et al, Prevention of colorectal cancer: guidelines based on new data. *WHO Bull OMS* 1995; **73:** 7–10.

23. Smith RA, von Eschenbach AC, Wender R et al, American Cancer Society guidelines for the early detection of cancer: update of early detection guidelines for prostate, colorectal and endometrial cancers. *CA Cancer J Clin* 2001; **51:** 38–75.

24. Winawer SJ, Fletcher RH, Miller L et al, Colorectal cancer screening: clinical guidelines and rationale. *Gastroenterology* 1997; **112:** 594–642.

25. Colorectal cancer screening. *Medicare Part B Newsletter* 1997; **155:** 2–3.

26. Anderson LM, May DS, Has the use of cervical, breast, and colorectal cancer screening increased in the United States? *Am J Public Health* 1995; **85:** 840–2.

27. Brown ML, Potosky AL, Thompson GB et al, The knowledge and use of screening tests for colorectal and prostate cancer: data from the 1987 National Health Interview Survey. *Prev Med* 1990; **19:** 562–7.

28. Centers for Disease Control and Prevention, Screening for colorectal cancer – United States, 1992–1993, and new guidelines. *MMWR* 1996; **45:** 107–10.

29. Lieberman D, Mass screening: North American perspective. In: *Prevention and Early Detection of Colorectal Cancer* (Young GP, Rozen P, Levin B, eds). London: Saunders, 1996: 289–300.

30. Speights VO, Johnson MW, Stoltenberg PH et al, Colorectal cancer: current trends in initial clinical manifestations. *South Med J* 1991; **84:** 575–8.

31. Majumdar SR, Fletcher RH, Evans AT, How does colorectal cancer present? Symptoms, duration, and clues to location. *Am J Gastroenterol* 1999; **94:** 3039–45.

32. Kyle SM, Isbister WH, Yeong ML. Presentation, duration of symptoms and staging of colorectal carcinoma. *Aust NZ J Surg* 1991; **61:** 137–40.

33. Lanier AP, Wychulis AR, Dockerty MB et al, Colorectal cancer in Rochester, Minnesota 1940–1969. *Cancer* 1973; **31:** 606–15.

34. Fijten GH, Starmans R, Muris JWM et al, Predictive value of signs and symptoms for colorectal cancer in patients with rectal bleeding in general practice. *Fam Pract* 1995; **12:** 279–286.

35. Metcalf JV, Smith J, Jones R et al, Incidence and causes of rectal bleeding in general practice as detected by colonoscopy. *Br J Gen*

Pract 1996; **46:** 161–4.

36. Norrelund N, Norrelund H, Colorectal cancer and polyps in patients aged 40 years and over who consult a GP with rectal bleeding. *Fam Pract* 1996; **13:** 160–5.

37. Rex DK, Colonoscopy: a review of its yield for cancers and adenomas by indication. *Am J Gastroenterol* 1995; **90:** 353–65.

38. Neugut AI, Garbowski GC, Waye JD et al. Diagnostic yield of colorectal neoplasia with colonoscopy for abdominal pain, change in bowel habits, and rectal bleeding. *Am J Gastroenterol* 1993; **88:** 1179–83.

39. Irvine EJ, O'Connor J, Frost RA et al, Prospective comparison of double contrast barium enema plus flexible sigmoidoscopy v colonoscopy in rectal bleeding: barium enema v colonoscopy in rectal bleeding. *Gut* 1988; **29:** 1188–93.

40. Jensen J, Kewenter J, Asztely M et al, Double contrast barium enema and flexible rectosigmoidoscopy: a reliable diagnostic combination for detection of colorectal neoplasm. *Br J Surg* 1990; **77:** 270–2.

41. Rex DK, Weddle RA, Lehman GA et al, Flexible sigmoidoscopy plus air contrast barium enema versus colonoscopy for suspected lower gastrointestinal bleeding. *Gastroenterology* 1990; **98:** 855–61.

42. Rex DK, Mark D, Clarke B et al, Flexible sigmoidoscopy plus air-contrast barium enema versus colonoscopy for evaluation of symptomatic patients without evidence of bleeding. *Gastrointest Endosc* 1995; **42:** 132–8.

2 What are the risk factors associated with colorectal cancer? An overview

Paul Rozen, Bernard Levin, Graeme P Young

Introduction

In Chapter 1, colorectal cancer has been identified as a worldwide major medical problem in 'westernized' countries (Figure 2.1).[1] For some decades, the USA, which is a high-incidence area, has recognized its public health importance. There, the incidence has recently shown a slight downturn, possibly because of the changes in lifestyle and dietary habits that have also reduced the incidence of cardiovascular disease. Mortality has also declined, mainly in US White women, and this reflects both its earlier diagnosis and improved therapy (see Figure 1.2 in Chapter 1). This high incidence is also found in those ethnically diverse and non-'Western' countries such as Japan, Singapore, and Israel, as well as the Czech Republic, etc., and occurs within one or two generations in immigrants moving from countries with a low colorectal cancer incidence to host countries of high incidence. From this, epidemiologists quickly concluded that acquired environmental and lifestyle factors must be the major etiological causes.[2]

The main environmental culprit was identified as being the Western-style diet, but, in addition, it was clear that, irrespective of diet, certain families were at risk for colorectal cancer. These two major etiologies of colorectal cancer – acquired and inherited – are discussed more fully in Chapters 4 and 6. This chapter will therefore be a synopsis of recognized risk factors and their relative contributions to the occurrence of colorectal cancer (Table 2.1). For simplicity, in this chapter, both colon and rectum, cancer and adenomatous polyps, are considered as one

Table 2.1 Genetic, dietary, lifestyle and past history risk factors and an estimation of their relative contributions to the occurrence of colorectal neoplasia

Risk factor	Minimal	Minor	Moderate	Major
Inherited, dominant				+
Inherited, recessive or low-penetrance			+	
Diet				+
Physical activity, decreased			+	
Frequent meals	+			
Gender, male		+		
Aging			+	
Obesity, body build		+		
Tobacco smoking		+		
Alcohol intake, chronic		+		
Laxative abuse, chronic	+			
Iron supplements, chronic	+			
Occupation	+			
Inflammatory bowel disease, chronic and extensive		+		
Acromegaly	+			
Diabetes mellitus	+			
Cholecystectomy	+			
Breast, ovarian cancer, radiation therapy		+		
Past colorectal cancer		+		
Past colorectal adenomatous polyp			+	

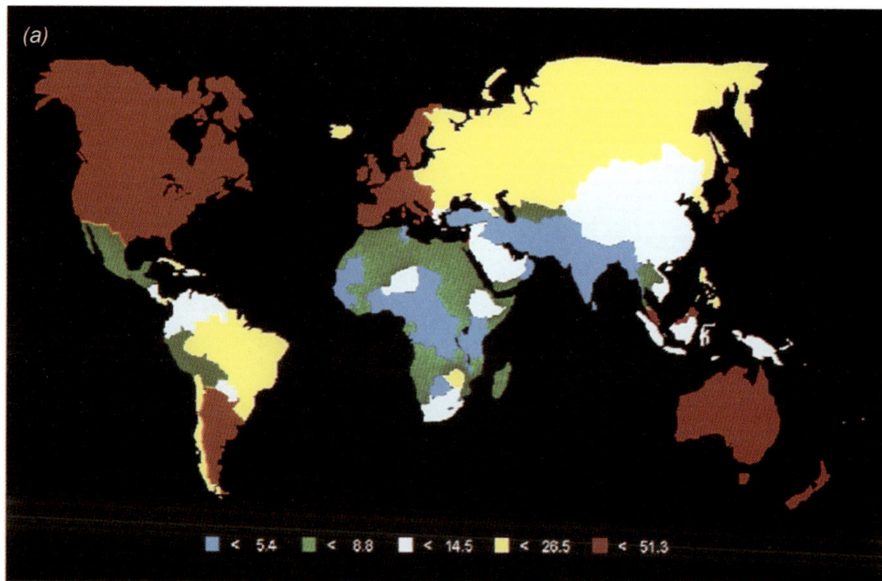

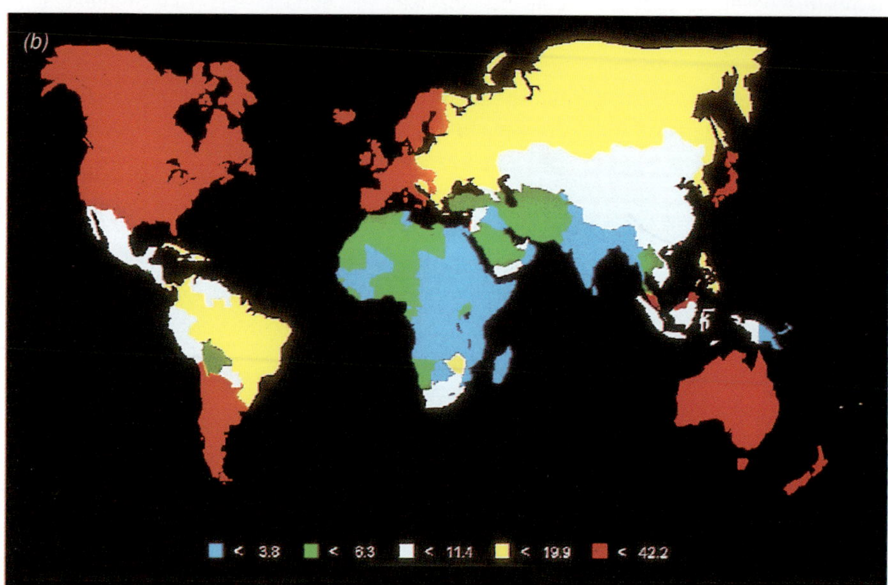

Figure 2.1 Worldwide range of colorectal cancer incidence, demonstrating the highest rates in countries having a 'westernized' lifestyle (age-standardized incidence): (a) males; (b) females. Prepared by Dr A Zauber, and derived from reference 1.

entity, although there are slight differences in epidemiology for each of them. It is clear that there is no one major environmental factor that explains all the risk for colorectal cancer, and extensive evidence points to the etiology of large-bowel neoplasia as being multifactorial. It may be easier to visualize the relationships of these etiological factors if we think of the 'stepwise' progression to cancer as follows: factors causing the expression of adenomatous tissue and polyp growth, factors causing progressive dysplasia, and factors allowing cancer to occur (Figure 2.2).

Major risk factors

Diet

A consistently high caloric intake leading to obesity, especially if associated with low physical activity, are both factors associated with risk for colorectal cancer. Eating frequent meals and thereby continuously promoting the flow of potentially carcinogenic bile salts has been associated with a higher risk for large-bowel cancer, but the evidence is tenuous.[2] Specific dietary risk factors include a *high* intake of animal fat and beef and eating it fried or charred. On the other hand, risk is also associated with a *low* intake of grains, fruits, and vegetables, which contain protective dietary fiber, minerals, vitamins, and bioactive compounds. Minerals such as calcium, found mainly in dairy products, are also protective, as is also an adequate fluid intake. For more details, see Chapter 4 and references therein.

Inherited risk factors

They include the defined genetic syndromes such as hereditary non-polyposis colorectal cancer, familial adenomatous polyposis, familial juvenile polyposis, and the Peutz–Jeghers syndrome. More common, but so far less well understood, is the familial clustering of colorectal and, or, other neoplasia, or the added risk of even having just a single first-degree relative with large-bowel cancer or adenomatous polyp. This is obviously a common occurrence, and probably points to the presence of a large pool of inherited genetic susceptibility factors in the general population.[2] These conditions are discussed in detail in Chapter 6.

Genetic–environmental interaction

It has been hypothesized that exposure to environmental risk factors, especially diet, can facilitate the clinical expression of recessive or low-penetrance inherited genetic etiologies of colorectal cancer, or influence the age at which it appears. This might explain why some cases of colorectal cancer occur within the generation of persons who migrated from low-incidence countries to high-incidence areas such as Australia or the USA.[2] Commonly occurring systemic (germline) genetic variations (polymorphisms) can influence the rates of detoxification or activation of environmental carcinogens (Table 2.2). These occur during the process of cooking, or from tobacco smoke, or alcohol metabolites, while there may be a lack of adequate amounts of dietary anticarcinogens, in the presence of an inability to metabolize these carcinogens.[2–4] This is an attractive explanation, but it is still uncertain that these genetic polymorphisms, i.e. minor variations in gene structure that do not lead to genetic disorders, represent a major contribution to the etiology of large-bowel neoplasia.

How much risk do these major factors contribute to colorectal neoplasia?

At present, we can conclude that the etiology of more than 30% of large-bowel neoplasia is related directly to the environment, namely diet and lifestyle of 'westernized' populations. It is estimated that the etiology of more than 15% is inherited and that the remainder are a result of an interaction between these etiologies[2–4] (Figure 2.3).

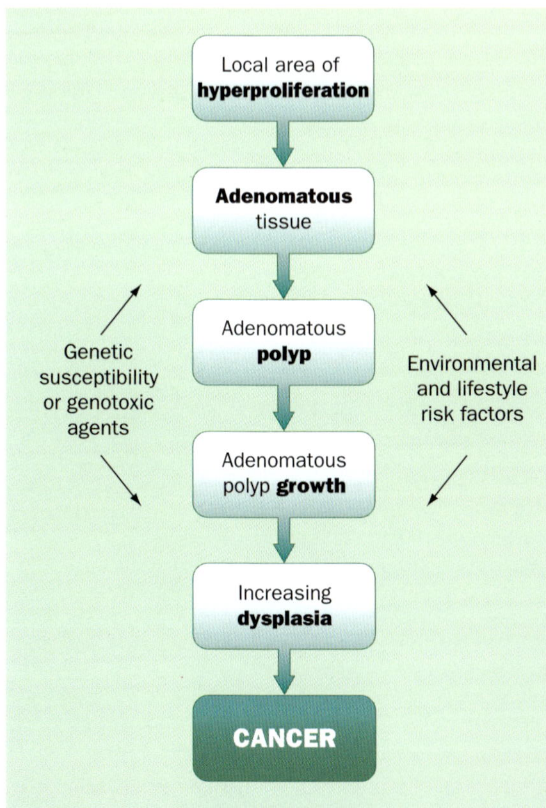

Figure 2.2 *Schematic representation of the stepwise progression with time, to adenoma, to increasing dysplasia, and finally to cancer.*

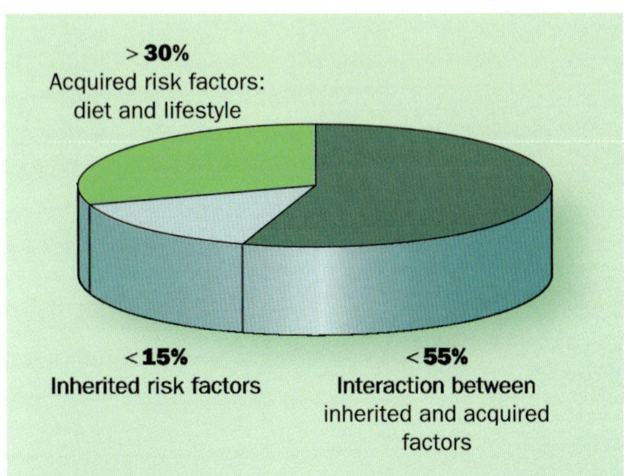

Figure 2.3 *Schematic representation of the relative contributions of acquired and inherited factors in the etiology of colorectal cancer and the possible interaction between them.*

Table 2.2 *Associations between environmental factors and metabolic phenotype in the etiology of colorectal neoplasia*[a]

Risk factor	Inadequate or disordered metabolic pathway	Result of perturbation
Red meat and high-temperature cooking	Acetylation of heterocyclic amines	Tumor induction
Fats, cholesterol	Apoprotein E	Chylomicron clearance Fecal bile acid output
Folate, methionine deficiency, alcohol	Methylation, thymidine synthesis	Mutation rates DNA strand breaks
Tobacco smoke	Glutathione conjugation, cytochrome enzyme AHH	DNA damage
Iron in meat, excessive intake	Hemochromatosis mutation	Excess free radicals

[a]Adapted from references 2 and 3.

Other known risk factors

The following have also been associated with risk for colorectal neoplasia. Even so, their quantitative contributions to the total burden of cancer are relatively small as compared with diet and genetic factors (Table 2.1).

Gender

As can be seen from Figure 2.4, on a country-to-country basis, the incidence of colorectal cancer is almost always higher in men than in women.[1] This difference is even greater for rectal cancer than for colon cancer.[1,2] These differences may be explained by different dietary and lifestyle habits, body build, physical activity, tobacco and

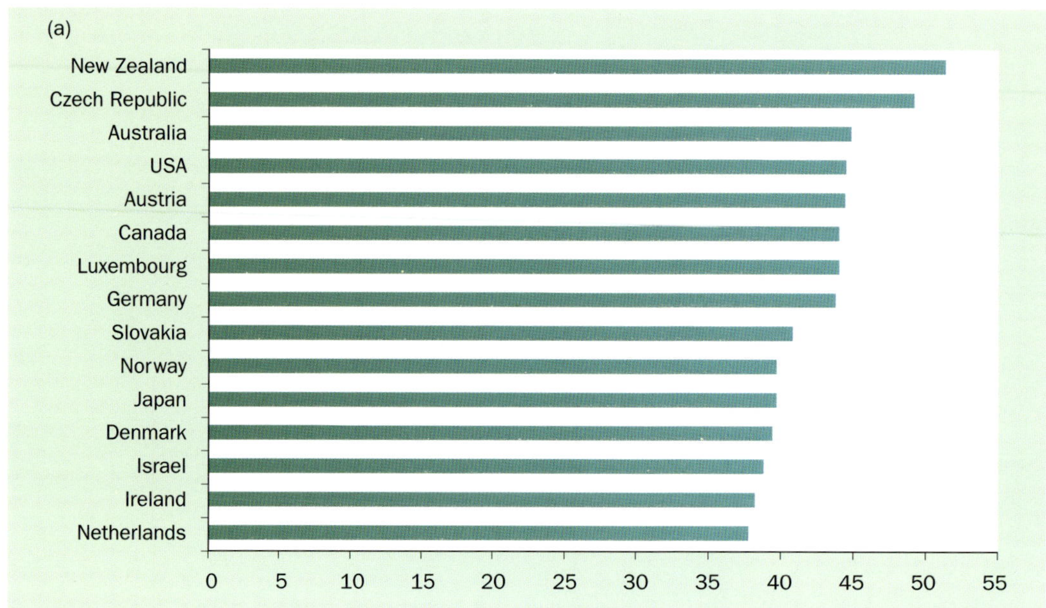

Figure 2.4 *Incidence, by country, of colorectal cancer (1990 age-standardized incidence per 100 000): (a,b) males; (c,d) females. Note that on a country-to-country basis, the incidence is higher in men. Prepared by Dr A Zauber, and derived from reference 1.*

alcohol use, consumption of non-steroidal anti-inflammatory drugs, and body stores of iron. There is also probably a protective effect associated with the female hormones and/or at least temporarily with the use of hormone replacement therapy (see Chapter 5).[2]

Age

The cumulative causes of colonic neoplastic changes (Figure 2.2) manifest themselves clinically as cancer in the later half of life (see Chapter 3). The incidence rises almost exponentially from the age of 50 years, and continues to rise dramatically for the duration of the population's lifespan (Figure 2.5). Mortality rates increase in parallel, at about 50% of the incidence, and show the same dramatic rise with aging.[5] For those reasons, early detection programs are initiated at the age of 50 years, and must be continued intensively throughout the life of healthy aging.

Body build

In addition to the cancer risk associated with excess weight, the body mass index, which takes into account

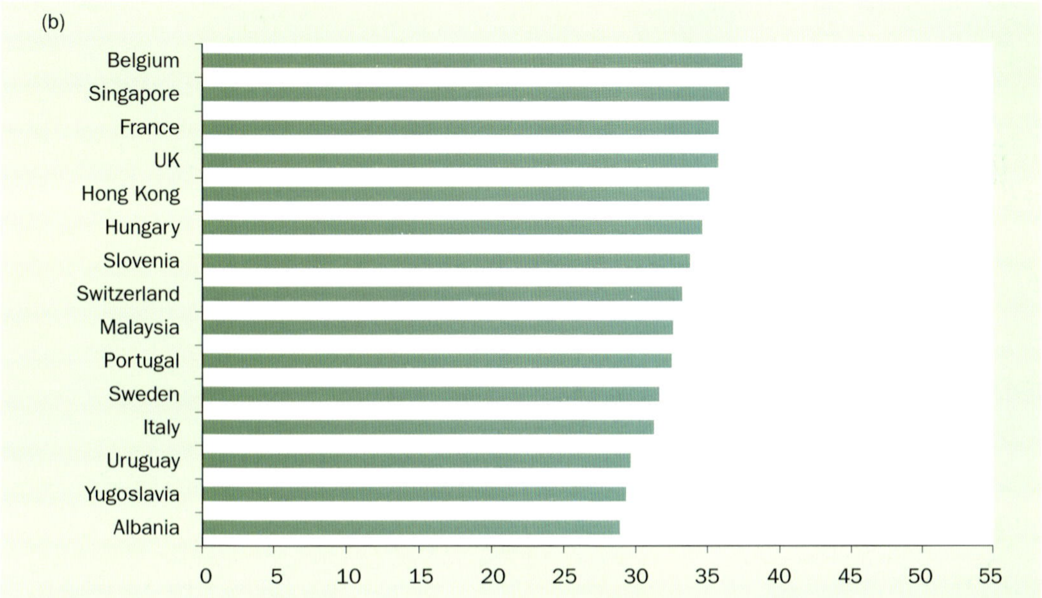

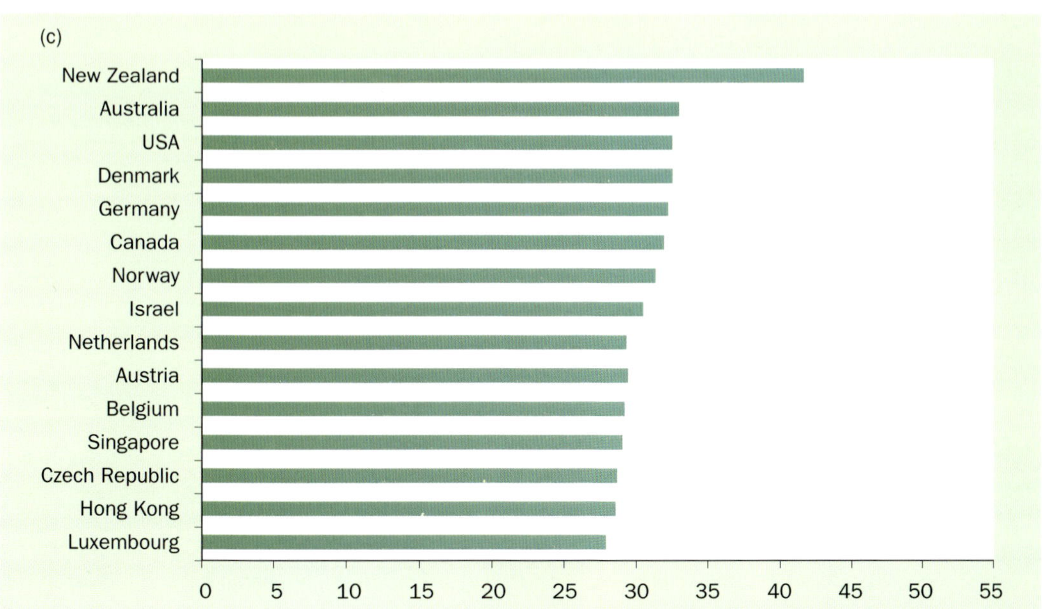

Continued

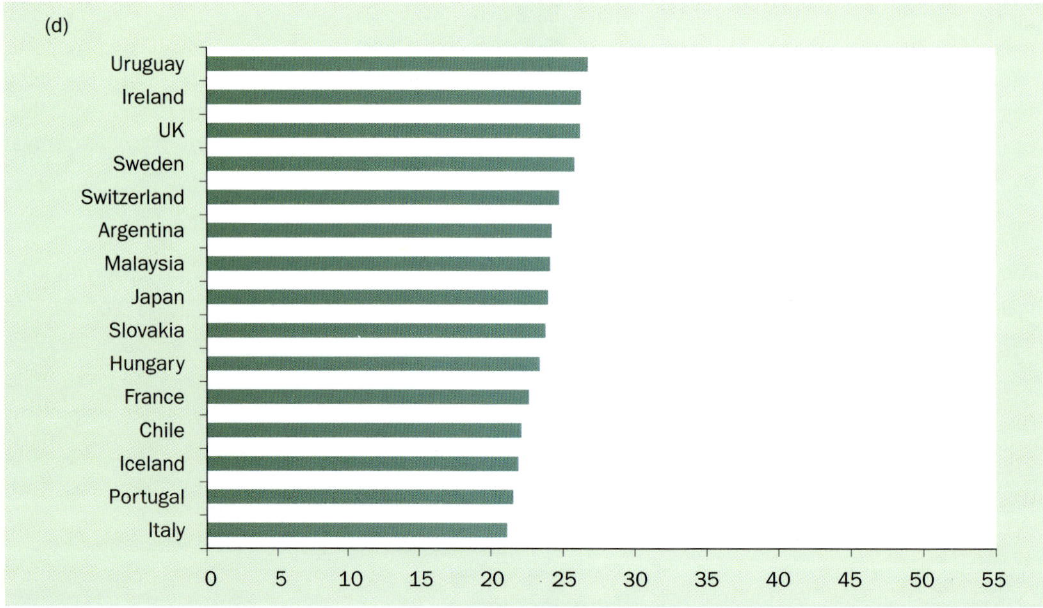

Figure 2.4 *(see page 18)*

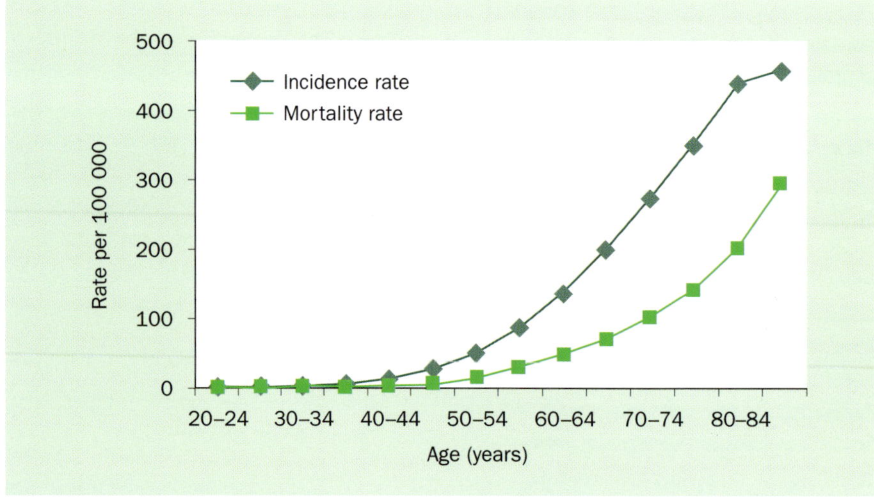

Figure 2.5 *Age-specific colorectal cancer incidence and mortality in the US general population, 1993–1997. Note the sharp rise in incidence and mortality with increasing age, after the age of 50 years. Prepared by Ms M Carlson and Dr A Zauber, and derived from reference 5.*

both height and weight (weight/height[2]), is also a risk factor for colorectal neoplasia.[2]

Tobacco smoking

The association is strongest for an increased prevalence of adenomas and less strong for risk of large-bowel cancer.[4] Even so, adenomas are potential precursors of cancers, and so tobacco smoking should also be considered in the etiology of colorectal cancer.

Alcohol

There is a weak association between alcohol consumption and risk for colon cancer.[6] The association is more consistent with rectal cancer, especially from beer drinking in most countries, but also for sake in Japan.[7] Murato et al[7] postulate that the acetaldehyde metabolite of alcohol causes DNA damage, and there are a number of Japanese who cannot detoxify this metabolite and are therefore genetically susceptible.

Laxative usage

In general, chronic constipation has not been regarded as a risk factor for colon neoplasia, although there are now some studies to indicate this possibility.[8] In addition, there are also some reports that have identified the chronic ingestion of phenolphthalein, and especially senna-containing laxatives, as being a minor risk factor for large-bowel epithelial hyperproliferation and even being associated with a risk for cancer.[9]

Iron supplements and hemochromatosis

To date, physicians have believed that for optimal health, the body stores of iron should be maintained full. There is some experimental and epidemiological evidence that chronic iron supplementation is a minor risk factor for cancer of various sites, including the large bowel.[10,11] The mechanism suggested is that unabsorbed dietary iron produces free radicals, which can cause mucosal damage.[11] A similar increased risk has also been noted to occur in persons found to be heterozygous for hereditary hemochromatosis, but who do not manifest the disease, a condition that is estimated to occur in 15% of the American population.[12]

Occupation

The only clear association of occupation with colorectal cancer is that of brewery workers who were given free access to their products.[2,4] There have been reports that asbestos workers were at slightly increased risk for colorectal neoplasia, but the overall evidence was not strong.[13] Today, because of public health measures preventing exposure to asbestos, this is not of clinical relevance.

Inflammatory bowel disease (IBD)

Chronic and extensive IBD, which leads to an increased turnover of epithelial cells, is associated with an increased risk for bowel cancer.[14] The risk is greater with ulcerative colitis than with Crohn's colitis. The longer the duration of disease (more than 8 years), and the more extensive the area of inflammation, more than the rectosigmoid, the greater the risk for cancer.[15] This is discussed more fully in Chapter 7.

Acromegaly

This uncommon disorder is due to the pituitary gland secreting an excessive amount of growth hormone. This condition has been found to be associated with a significant risk for both colorectal adenomas and cancer.[16,17]

Diabetes mellitus

A very large epidemiological survey of diabetic patients showed that they had a slightly increased risk for colorectal cancer.[18]

Cholecystectomy

Several large population studies of women post cholecystectomy confirmed that they are at slightly increased risk for right-sided colon cancer, 15 or more years after surgery.[19] This has been explained by the constant free entry of bile into that site.

Breast and ovarian cancer, radiation therapy

Women who survive a breast or ovarian malignancy are at a slightly increased risk, about 1.5–2 times that expected, to develop a large-bowel malignancy.[20–22] The risk is probably related to unrecognized inherited risk factors and/or common etiological dietary and lifestyle causes.[21,22] A similar, slightly increased risk for colorectal cancer can also be found in first-degree relatives of breast cancer patients.[20] In the case of ovarian cancer, radiation therapy may have contributed to the appearance of rectal cancer.[22,23]

Past colorectal cancer or adenomatous polyp

Metachronous large-bowel cancer can appear in persons after successful surgery for a colorectal cancer. This is a lifetime risk, and has been calculated as being 0.35% per year.[24] Similarly, persons who have had an adenomatous polyp are at risk for further polyps. This risk is least in persons having had a single small tubular adenoma without high-grade dysplasia, and there is an increased risk if the adenomatous polyps were large, sessile, multiple, villous, or showed high-grade dysplasia, and if there was a family history of colorectal neoplasia.[25] See Chapter 7 for more details.

Conclusions

From the above review, it can be seen that many conditions are associated with a slightly increased risk for colorectal cancer (Table 2.1). However, their individual overall contributions to the total cancer burden are small. One must not lose sight that of the two most important etiologies that we know about, one is acquired – diet and lifestyle – and the other is inherited – susceptibility. Prevention, therefore, is aimed at recognizing this susceptibility, correcting acquired risk habits, and detecting treatable neoplasia early on.

References (*Reviews and general articles)

1. Parkin DM, Pisani P, Ferlay J, Estimates of the worldwide incidence of 25 major cancers in 1990. *Int J Cancer* 1999; **80**: 827–41.

2. *Potter JD, Epidemiologic, environmental and lifestyle issues in colorectal cancer. In: *Prevention and Early Detection of Colorectal Cancer* (Young GP, Rozen P, Levin B, eds). London: Saunders, 1996: 23–43.

3. *Gertig DN, Hunter DJ, Genes and environment in the etiology of colorectal cancer. *Semin Cancer Biol* 1998; **8**: 285–98.

4. Terry MB, Neugut AI, Cigarette smoking and the colorectal adenoma–carcinoma sequence: a hypothesis to explain the paradox. *Am J Epidemiol* 1998; **147**: 903–10.

5. Ries LAG, Eisner MP, Kosary CL et al (eds), *SEER Cancer Statistics Review, 1973–1997*. Bethesda, MD: National Cancer Institute, 2000. http://seer.cancer.gov/ Publications/CSR1973_1997/.

6. *Kune GA, Vitetta L, Alcohol consumption and the etiology of colorectal cancer: a review of the scientific evidence from 1957 to 1991 (Review). *Nutr Cancer* 1992; **18**: 97–111.

7. Murato M, Tagawa M, Watanabe S et al, Genotype difference of aldehyde dehydrogenase 2 gene in alcohol drinkers influences the incidence of Japanese colorectal cancer patients. *Jpn J Cancer Res* 1999; **90**: 711–19.

8. Jacobs EJ, White E, Constipation, laxative use and colon cancer among middle-aged adults. *Epidemiology* 1998; **9**: 385–91.

9. *van Gorkom BAAP, de Vries EGE, Karrenbeldd A et al, Anthranoid laxatives and their potential carcinogenic effects (Review). *Aliment Pharmacol Ther* 1999; **13**: 443–52.

10. *Stevens RG, Jones Y, Micozzi MS et al, Body iron stores and the risk of cancer. *N Engl J Med* 1988; **319**: 1047–52.

11. Lund EK, Wharf SG, Fairweather-Tait SJ et al, Oral ferrous sulfate supplements increase the free radical-generating capacity of feces from healthy volunteers. *Am J Clin Nutr* 1999; **69**: 250–5.

12. Nelson RL, Davis FG, Persky V et al, Risk of neoplastic and other diseases among people with heterozygosity for hereditary hemochromatosis. *Cancer* 1995; **76**: 875–9.

13. Gamble JF, Asbestos and colon cancer: a weight-of-the-evidence review. *Environ Health Perspect* 1994; **102**: 1038–50.

14. *Goldman H, Significance and detection of dysplasia in chronic colitis (editorial). *Cancer* 1996; **78**: 2261–3.

15. Persson P-G, Bernell O, Leijonmarck C-E et al, Survival and cause-specific mortality in inflammatory bowel disease: a population-based cohort study. *Gastroenterology* 1996; **110**: 1339–45.

16. Ron E, Gridley G, Hrubec Z et al, Acromegaly and gastrointestinal cancer. *Cancer* 1991; **68**: 1673–7.

17. Delhougne B, Deneux C, Abs R et al, The prevalence of colonic polyps in acromegaly: a colonoscopic and pathological study in 103 patients. *J Clin Endocrinol Metab* 1995; **80**: 3223–6.

18. Will JC, Galuska A, Vinicor F et al, Colorectal cancer: another complication of diabetes mellitus? *Am J Epidemiol* 1998; **147**: 816–25.

19. Ekbom A, Yuen J, Adami H-O et al, Cholecystectomy and colorectal cancer. *Gastroenterology* 1993; **105**: 142–7.

20. Howell MA, The association between colorectal cancer and breast cancer. *J Chron Dis* 1976; **29**: 243–61.

21. Rozen P, Hallak A, Rozen S et al, The value of screening women for large bowel tumors after breast or reproductive organ cancer. *Front Gastrointest Res* 1986; **10**: 206–15.

22. Travis LB, Curtis RE, Boice, JD Jr et al, Second malignant neoplasms among long-term survivors of ovarian cancer. *Cancer Res* 1996; **56**: 1564–70.

23. Boice, JD Jr, Day NE, Andersen A et al, Second cancers following radiation treatment for cervical cancer. An international collaboration among cancer registries. *J Natl Cancer Inst* 1985; **74**: 955–75.

24. Cali RL, Pitsch PM, Thorson AAG et al, Cumulative incidence of metachronous colorectal cancer. *Dis Colon Rectum* 1993; **36**: 388–93.

25. *Bochud M, Burnand B, Froehlich F et al, Appropriateness of colonoscopy: surveillance after polypectomy. *Endoscopy* 1999; **31**: 654–63.

How does colorectal cancer develop?

Graeme P Young, Paul Rozen, Bernard Levin

Introduction

The process of development of colorectal cancer involves interactions between the genome (the genetic components) of the colorectal epithelial cell and its environment.[1] These interactions are shown conceptually in Figure 3.1. Both inherent genetic and externally determined environmental factors are important causes of tumorigenesis (the process of development of a tumor).[1,2] The colonic lumenal environment is complex, and is subject to great variability, largely due to diet. As a consequence, dietary lifestyle is very important.[2] This accounts for the characteristic international epidemiology of this disease, where colorectal cancer is more common in countries that follow, or are moving towards, a Western dietary lifestyle.[2]

The basic biology of gastrointestinal neoplasia is complex, and involves concepts such as tumor genetics, multistage carcinogenesis, oncogene activation, tumor suppressor gene inactivation, expansion of clones of neoplastic cells, homeostatic control of tumor growth, and cell invasion. The purpose of this chapter is to provide a simplified presentation of these concepts to aid understanding of their relevance to primary prevention, early detection, and overall clinical management, including definition of risk.

The characteristics of a cancer cell

Normal cellular control mechanisms involve four key biological processes,[3] as conceptualized in Figure 3.2:

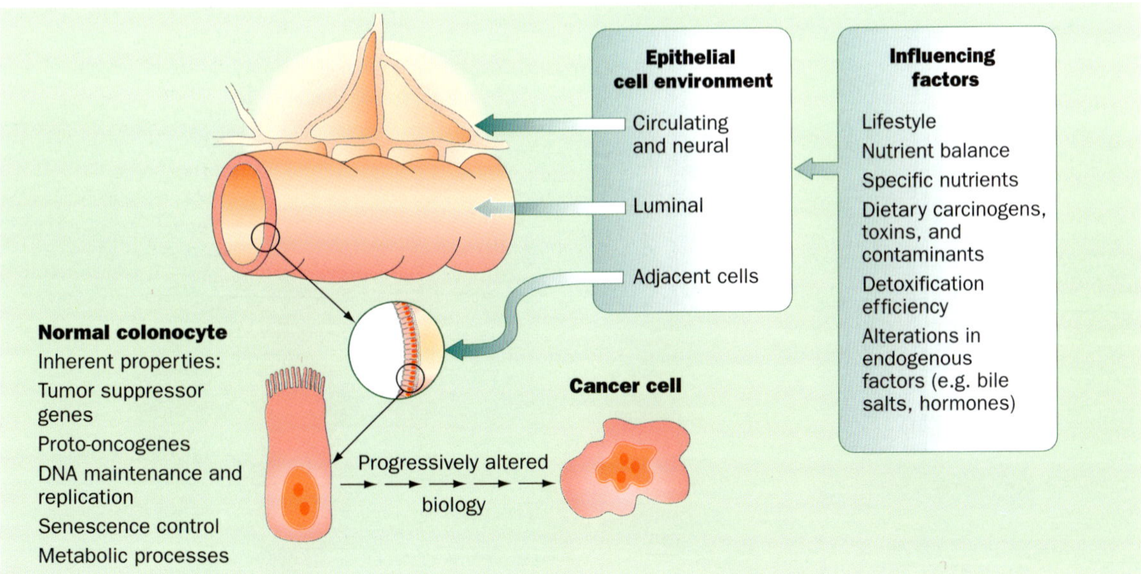

Figure 3.1 *Conceptual representation of interactions between the colonic epithelial cell and its environment. Influencing factors that regulate the processes leading to tumorigenesis may be endogenous or exogenous in origin, and sometimes endogenous but with exogenous influences (e.g. dietary fats on bile salts). The epithelial environment is complex, with many variables and influencing agents acting via the lumen. The cell is not a passive target, and contains inherent protective processes, which need to be disordered or overwhelmed before the progressively altered biology of tumorigenesis is set in motion.*

(i)   cell proliferation regulated by checkpoints in the cell cycle;

(ii) cell death regulated by an inherent cellular process called programmed cell death or apoptosis;

(iii) cell relationships with the immediate environment, i.e. cell–cell and intracellular signaling pathways;

(iv) cell position, i.e. its anchorage to basement membrane.

Cell birth and death (collectively often referred to simply as growth), relationship to environment, and cell locale become disturbed in a cancer cell.

Proliferation: cell-cycle checkpoints

The cycle of cell replication consists of five phases. The total duration varies from 12 to 48 hours, depending on conditions, with the variability being due to changes in duration of G_1 (the resting phase). In the crypt, its proliferative compartment (the lowest one-fifth), 10–20% of the cells have the potential for DNA synthesis and chromosomal duplication (S phase) at any one time. They then go into G_2, which is preparation for cell division, then mitosis, which is M phase. Following this, the cells then go back to G_1 and a controlled proportion of cells leave G_1 for G_0, which is terminal differentiation, and eventual apoptosis (cell death). Various cell-cycle checkpoint proteins regulate this ordered process, but in cancer cells, the checkpoints become disordered, with the result that proliferation may no longer be controlled.

Apoptosis: programmed cell death

Programmed cell death, or apoptosis, is a physiologic process essential for normal tissue turnover, deletion of genetically damaged cells, and embryonic development.[4] By this process, a cell dies owing to internal activation of nucleus-destroying enzymes. It is irreversible, and ensures that cells do not become immortal or pass genetic abnormalities on to their progeny. In the colon, apoptosis controls the rate of growth and prevents undue expansion of the proliferative compartment situated towards the base of the crypt (see Figure 3.3). In cancers, the mechanisms controlling apoptosis, which are dependent in part on proteins coded by the *APC* and the *bcl-2* gene family, become disordered and uncontrolled,[5] and genetically damaged cells may be able to survive and replicate. Overexpression of cyclooxygenase-2 confers resistance to normal apoptotic control.

Cell relationships and signaling

Gastrointestinal epithelium requires neighboring cells to form a tight barrier; this is achieved by cell–cell adhesion at the zona adherens. Normal complexing between the APC protein, E-cadherin, and β-catenin ensures normal cell–cell interaction, growth control, and maturity of cell function. In cancers, a variety of molecular disturbances, including mutation of the *APC* and *β-catenin* genes, disrupt

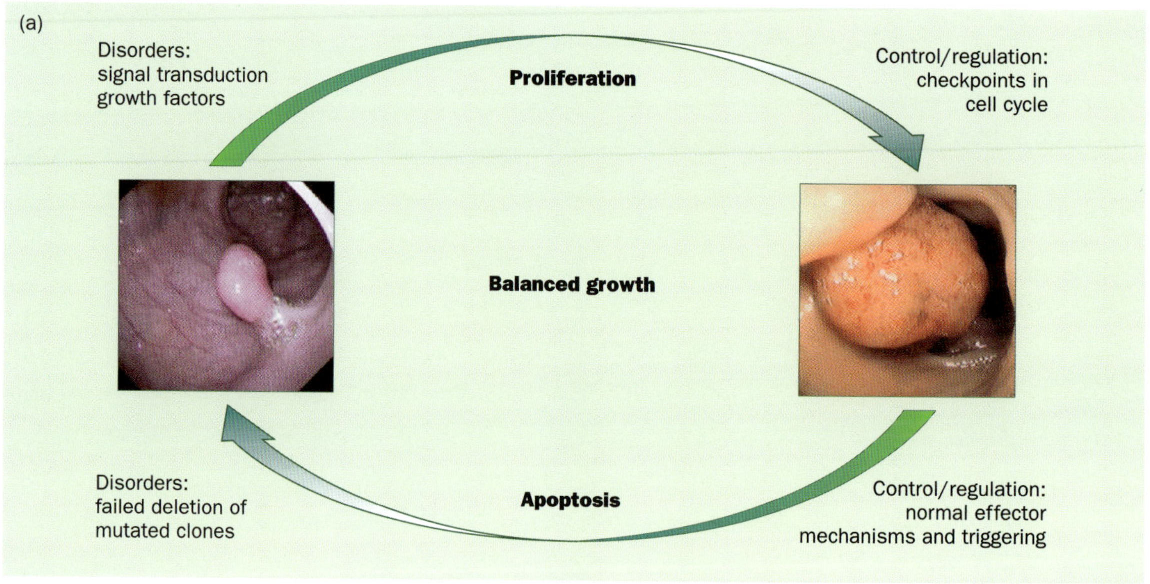

Figure 3.2 *Main biological processes inherent in control of cellular normality. (a) Concepts in the control of growth.*

this complexing, with resultant disturbances in growth control and function.[6]

Interaction between epithelial and other mucosal cells is also important. Growth factors originating from neigh-boring (paracrine) cells, bind to a receptor on the epithelial cell and modulate growth characteristics. Binding activates intracellular signaling pathways. This process of signal transduction becomes disordered in a variety of ways in cancer.[3] In some instances (e.g. mutation of the K-*ras* oncogene), the signaling pathway becomes continually and uncontrollably activated, and growth is no longer effectively regulated. Other similar disorders occur, such as with transforming growth factor β1 (TGF-β1) and its receptor.

Cell anchorage to the basement membrane

In the colon, the essential difference between the benign precancer epithelial lesion (i.e. dysplasia) and cancer is the loss of anchorage of the cell to its basement mem-brane.[3] This enables passage of the cell through the base-ment membrane, i.e. local invasion. Loss of normal basement-membrane anchorage and secretion of invasion-mediating enzymes such as urokinase are vital biological characteristics of the cancer cell.

Cancer cell biology and its acquisition

A neoplastic colonic epithelial cell is characterized by various combinations of the above biological aberrations (Figure 3.2). For such biological processes to become deranged, changes in the genetic make-up of the cell must occur.[7] Not all changes will occur at once or necessarily within a short timeframe. Understanding how a colorectal cancer develops thus involves an understanding about

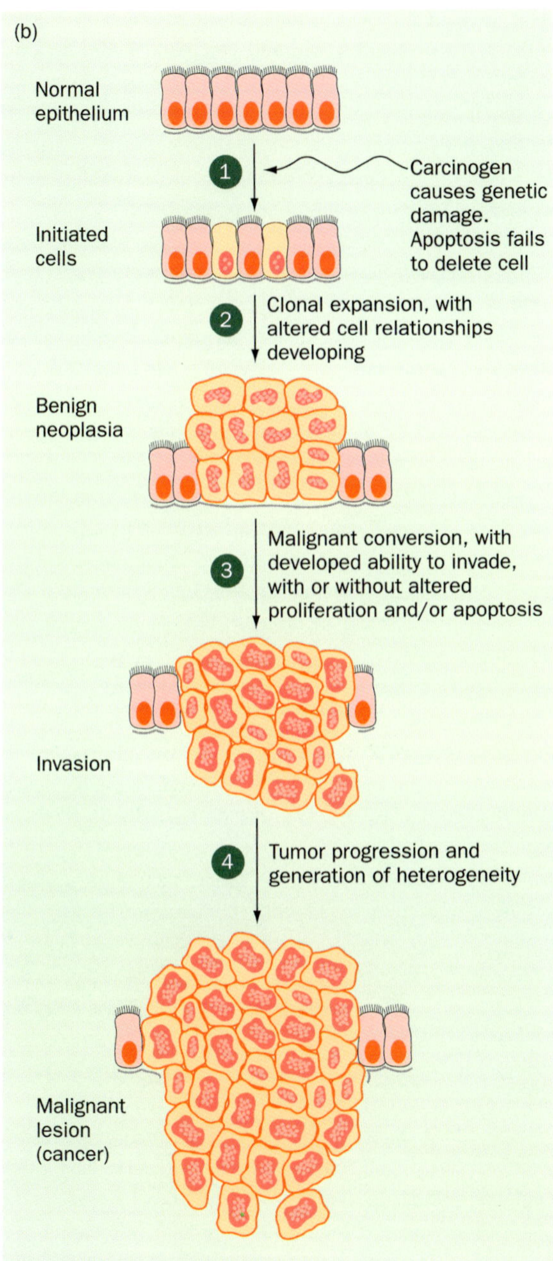

Figure 3.2 *continued.*
(b) Concepts of morphological progression through tumorigenesis, incorporating altered cell relationships and invasion through the basement membrane. Adapted from reference 3, with permission from the publishers Lippincott Williams and Wilkins.

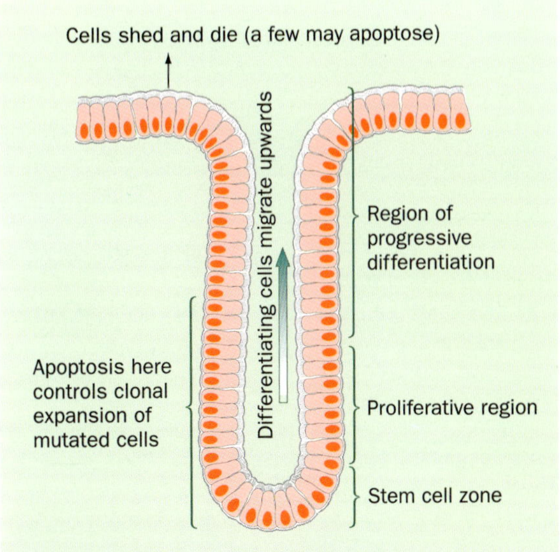

Figure 3.3 *Epithelial compartments of the normal colonic crypt, demonstrating the proliferative and differentiation compartments and showing how apoptosis will prevent expansion of mutated clones.*

how these biological changes come about, the time-frame over which they occur, and the mechanisms by which they might be regulated, especially by external influences.

Models of colorectal cancer development

Cancer can be considered to be an acquired genetic disease, sometimes with inherited genetic factors making a contribution, resulting from exposure over many years to environmental carcinogens and other regulators.[8]

Tumorigenesis in the colon and rectum was initially described in terms of the classic 'initiation–promotion model'.[1,3] In this model, the first step involves direct damage to DNA, which resulted in mutations, i.e. 'initiation'. Surviving mutated cells proliferate, and if the mutations are biologically significant, then this eventually progresses through to cancer, driven to completion by promotional factors that in themselves do not necessarily damage DNA but do modify biological responsiveness. The initiation and promotion processes were conceived of as being strictly sequential.

The multistep model of colorectal tumorigenesis
A new model termed 'multistep carcinogenesis' appears to provide a better explanation of tumorigenesis.[1,3] The process is largely driven by mutations and other genetic abnormalities, randomly occurring at different points in time, at multiple sites on DNA. It could be thought of as multiple, superimposed, initiation–promotion models, but this would not adequately allow for the biological complexity of the new model.[1]

Inherent in the multistep model of tumorigenesis are two important molecular genetic concepts:

1. The genome of the cell becomes progressively unstable during tumorigenesis.
2. Abnormalities occur in genes that are critical in maintaining the non-neoplastic phenotype.

Genomic stability is maintained by what may be termed *caretaker* genes.[7] Abnormalities in these increase the likelihood that further genetic abnormalities will occur. If, by chance, an abnormality arises in a gene with a fundamentally important biological role, then a function important for the neoplastic phenotype may be acquired. These normal genes are *gatekeepers*.[7]

Exposure to environmental agents is episodic and cumulative, although probably frequent. The resultant

mutations give rise to the multistep process, spread over a considerable time during which these chance events accumulate. No single genetic mutation is so critical to the process that it alone will result in cancer, although certain mutations may be inherited that accelerate the process. At some point, genomic instability gives rise to spontaneous genetic abnormalities without the need for additional carcinogen-induced mutations.

Conceptualized from the biological perspective, tumorigenesis begins with mutations in critical growth-regulating genes that either result in enhanced proliferation (loss of normal controls of proliferation) or prevention of death by apoptosis (loss of immortality-preventing factors). Cells that survive with these mutations may have a growth and survival advantage and so displace the neighboring normal cells through successive waves of cellular clonal expansion and selection. With time, a subclone may acquire the full malignant phenotype (see Figure 3.2). Eventually, further biological changes may occur that confer metastatic capacities.

Cell phenotype progressively changes, first with the formation of dysplasia and later the evolution of carcinoma, i.e. the adenoma–carcinoma sequence (Figure 3.4). The likelihood of accumulating such events increases with time such that cancer incidence rises as an exponential function of age.

The adenoma–carcinoma sequence
The concept of cancer development via benign neoplasms characterized as adenomatous polyps has progressively gained creditability over almost three decades.[9] While sometimes called the polyp–cancer sequence, this is technically incorrect in that 'polyp' simply describes a shape and need not refer to an early neoplasm. The key morphological hallmark of neoplasia in an adenoma is dysplasia.[10] Dysplasia is characterized by progressive cytologic and architectural abnormalities, but the cells are not invasive. Adenoma tissue does not always take on the shape of polyps, and hence a more correct term would be 'dysplasia–carcinoma' sequence.

While most colorectal carcinomas arise one way or another from dysplastic epithelium, it is also clear that most adenomas do not develop into carcinomas.[11] The exact frequency and time course of this neoplastic progression is not clearly defined, because for ethical reasons polyps once identified are removed, but predictions can be made based on observational studies. The peak age at which adenomas develop is 50 years, and precedes the peak age of development of carcinomas by about 7 years.[12] This suggests that adenomas progress over a period of 5–10 years before becoming cancers (Figure 3.5).

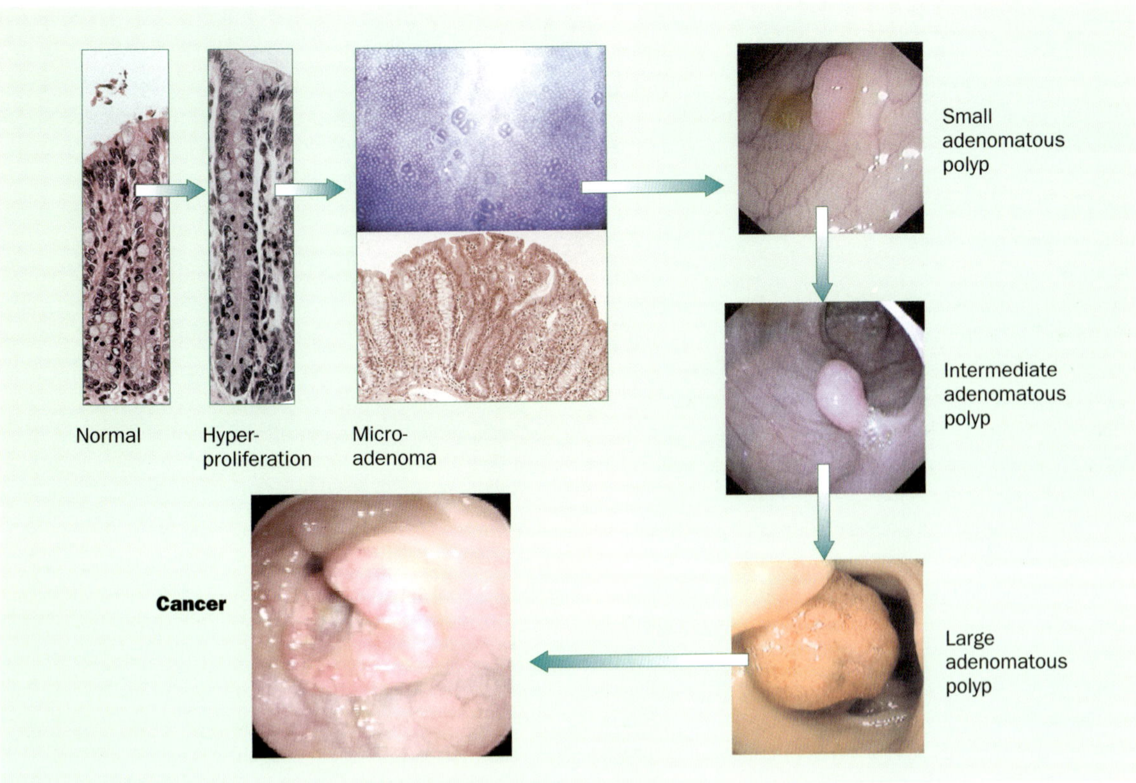

Figure 3.4 *Phenotypic stages in the adenoma–carcinoma sequence. Note that the hallmark of the adenoma is dysplasia. Strictly speaking, this represents the premalignant lesion, since dysplastic tissue might not take on the form of a polyp (i.e. it may remain a flat adenoma).*

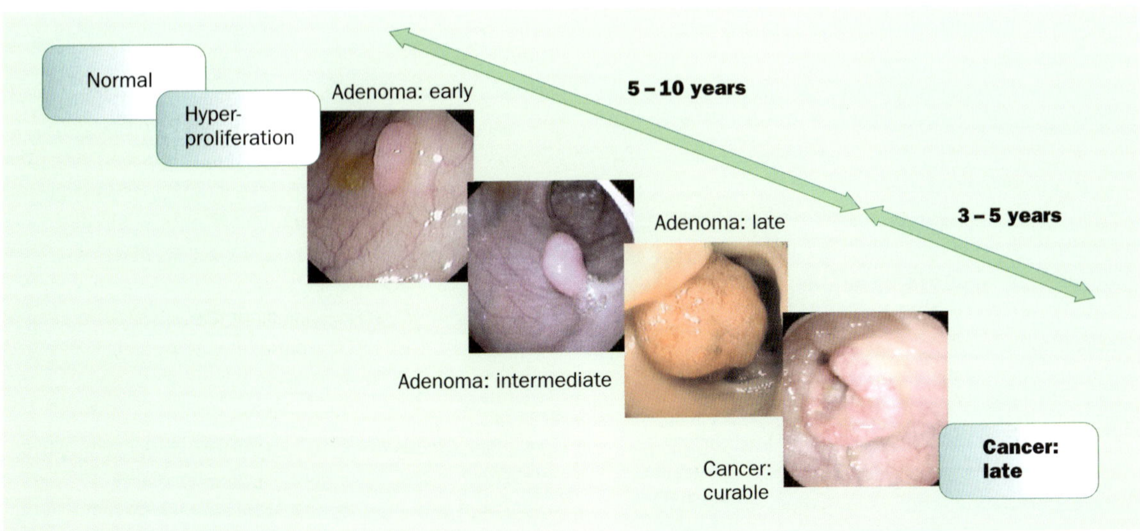

Figure 3.5 *Time course of sporadic colorectal cancer development in the human colon. Figures 3.7 and 3.8 show the alternative pathways for the dominantly inherited cancer syndromes. Progression is characterized by increasing adenoma size, amount of villous histology, dysplasia, and often multiple numbers of polyps.*

Evidence for the adenoma–carcinoma sequence

The evidence for the adenoma–carcinoma sequence is derived from epidemiological, morphologic, biological, anecdotal clinical, and therapeutic data. There is a close association between adenomas and carcinomas.[1] For instance, 30% of patients with colorectal cancer have at least one synchronous adenoma, and in those with two or more synchronous cancers, 50–85% have a synchronous adenoma.

While it is ethically difficult to leave adenomas untreated, the available evidence suggests that progression to cancer does occur. Cancers have been found to develop at the site of adenomas left untreated because of patient non-compliance or technical difficulties. Additional evidence comes from studies involving the detection and removal of adenomatous polyps. For instance, in a large study, the frequency of carcinomas occurring in the 7–14 years subsequent to polypectomy was about a third of the expected rate in an untreated population.[13]

The term 'de novo' or 'in situ' tumorigenesis has emerged in the last few years to cover the concept that a cancer did not develop from a macroscopically obvious adenomatous polyp.[14] The possibility that a dysplastic lesion does not precede the invasive-cancer phenotype, however, seems unlikely. Small colorectal carcinomas normally arise in adenomas, whereas small carcinomas not associated with adenomas are relatively rare in Western countries. Recent observations in Japan and Europe, however, indicate that a sizeable *minority* of cancers do develop without recognizable adenomatous co-pathology.

Overview of genetic events associated with tumorigenesis

With progression of adenomas to carcinomas, there is a progressive accumulation of genetic abnormalities consistent with the multistep model. The biological significance of these is discussed in a subsequent section, but the following is a brief synopsis of the timing of abnormalities in the common gatekeeper genes in tumorigenesis. These events are summarized in Figure 3.6.

1. The most prevalent molecular genetic abnormality in the earliest neoplastic pathology identifiable – termed aberrant crypt foci or microadenomas (i.e. dysplastic crypts) – is that of mutations in the *ras* proto-oncogene.[15] These mutations are passed to subsequent expanding clones, since about half of colorectal adenomas and cancers have been found to have *K-ras* gene mutations.

2. Mutations in the *APC* gene, found on chromosome 5, appear to be an early event associated with small-adenoma development and epithelial hyperproliferation, although the precise point in progression varies between those with sporadic cancers and those with FAP (familial adenomatous polyposis).[16] Not only are mutations in the *APC* gene responsible for FAP, but abnormalities are also common in sporadic colon carcinomas, where they are obviously acquired rather than inherited.

3. Loss of chromosomal alleles is observed in larger adenomas. Allelic losses of chromosomes 5 (the mechanism for altered *APC* in sporadic cancers) and/or of chromosome 18 (site of the *DCC* gene), are progressively common in larger adenomas and cancers.[17]

4. A pivotal event associated with transition from dysplasia to the cancer phenotype is loss of function of the p53 protein, whose gene is found on chromosome 17.[18]

How do mutations and other genetic abnormalities arise?

Mutations in the genome are either inherited or acquired. Those that are acquired may be due to chance mutations occurring as part of the normal cellular life span (see below), or else may be related to dietary lifestyle (Table 3.1).

Inherited mutations

Inherited mutations may be direct and powerful, such as mutations of the *APC* gene responsible for FAP or of the DNA mismatch-repair genes (see below) responsible for hereditary non-polyposis colorectal cancer (HNPCC), or they may be indirect and less powerful, such as the genes that control metabolism of dietary procarcinogens. These are represented schematically in Figures 3.7 and 3.8. Further details of the inherited syndromes are given in Chapter 6.

Acquired mutations and genomic abnormalities

Damage can occur to normal cellular genes through a variety of spontaneous and induced mechanisms. Mutations may be spontaneous due to the instability of the purine and pyrimidine bases themselves and lead to mispairing during the next round of replication. DNA-repair systems normally correct these.[19]

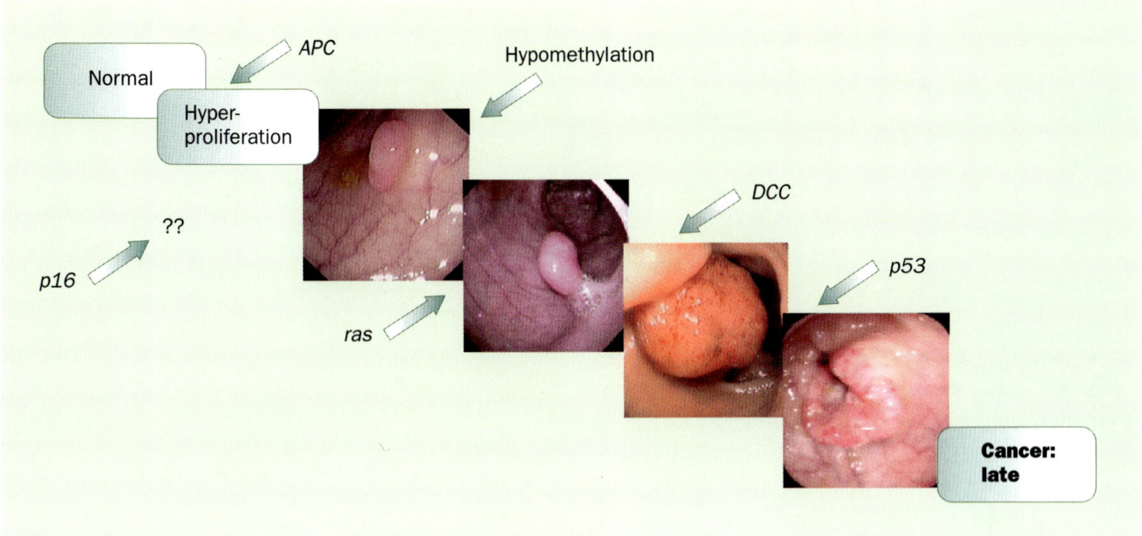

Figure 3.6 *Main molecular events in the development of sporadic colorectal cancers. Not all cancers possess each of these, although when this is the case, mutations in or deletions of other genes with similar functions are thought to occur. The nature of the molecular abnormalities in these genes varies with the situation, and is discussed briefly in the text.*

Table 3.1 *Process of occurrence of mutations and other genetic abnormalities relevant to colorectal cancer*

Process	Examples of process
Inherited	● Tumor suppressor genes: *APC* ● DNA mismatch-repair genes: *MLH1, MSH2*, etc. ● Carcinogen-metabolizing genes: *NAT1, NAT2*, etc.
Acquired ● Spontaneous due to base instability: causes point mutations ● Induced by carcinogens: causes point mutations ● DNA rearrangement: due to progressively unstable genome ● DNA deletion: due to progressively unstable genome ● DNA amplification ● DNA hypomethylation	● Tumor suppressor genes: *APC, p53, DCC* ● Oncogenes: *ras, myc, myb* ● Cell-cycle checkpoints: *p16*

Several environmental factors predictably induce damage to DNA, including viral infections, chemical carcinogens, and radiation (ionizing radiation such as X-rays and γ-rays, and particle radiation such as electrons, α-particles, and heavy ions). With colorectal cancer, viral infections and radiation are rare causes, but dietary chemical carcinogens are important because of the direct exposure of the gut.

Chemical carcinogenesis

Chemical carcinogens are ubiquitous in the human diet, and studies have demonstrated increased mutagenic activity in the stools of patients at risk for colorectal neoplasia.[20] Typically, carcinogens occur in foods in forms that need to be activated (i.e. procarcinogens), and are modified by metabolic processes in the liver and colonic mucosa to either activate or deactivate them. The microbial flora of the gastrointestinal tract and certain phytochemicals (bioactive components of plants) are also important in their activation and deactivation.[21]

Carcinogen metabolism

There are large individual differences in cancer susceptibility. In colorectal cancer, evidence points to an

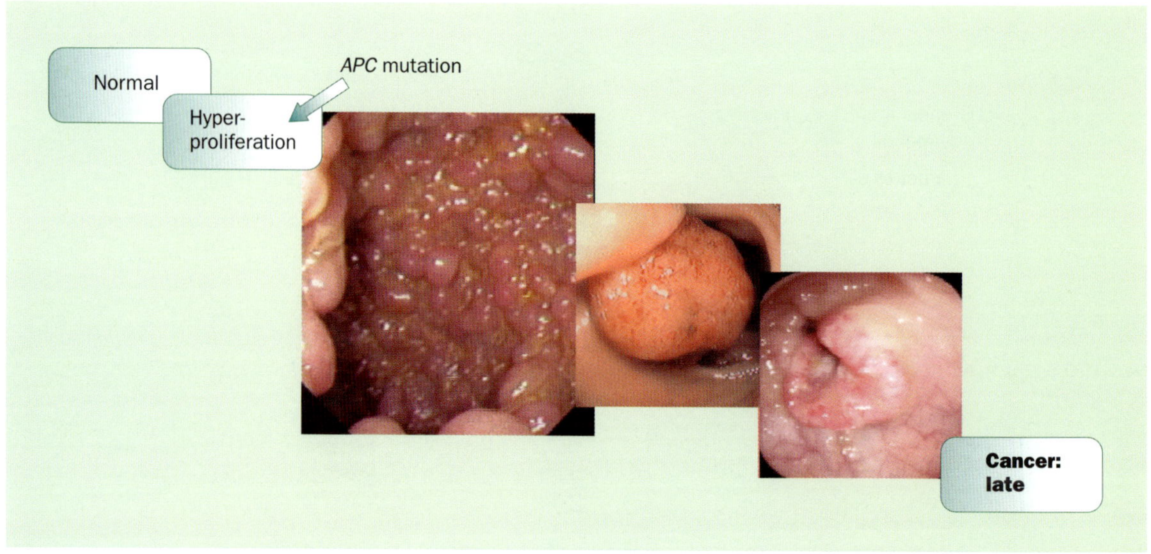

Figure 3.7 *Schematic representation of tumorigenesis in familial adenomatous polyposis (FAP). The early development of massive numbers of adenomatous polyps is the key biological change.*

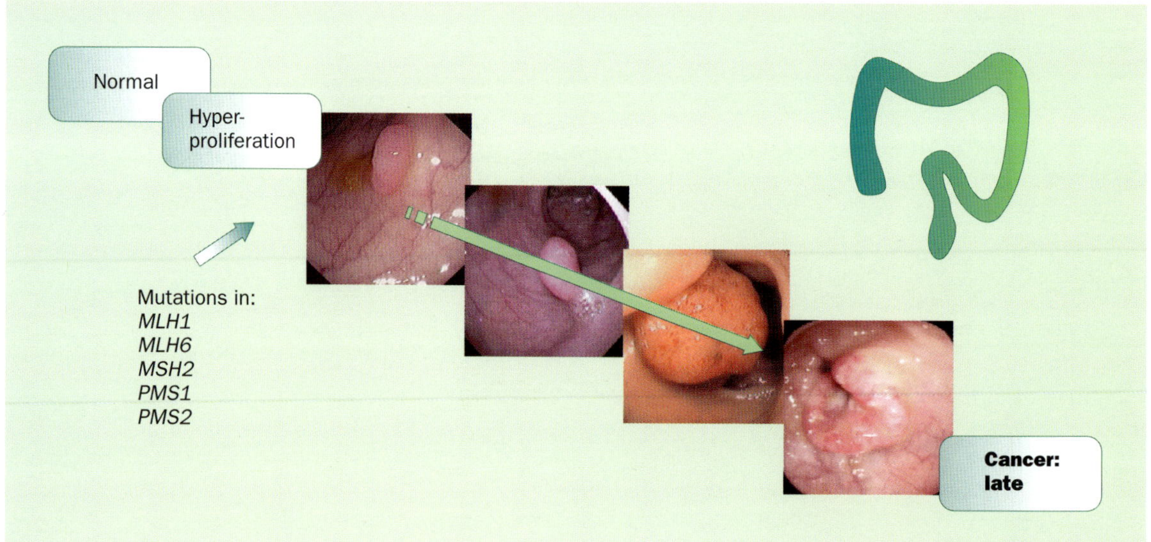

Figure 3.8 *Schematic representation of tumorigenesis in hereditary non-polyposis colorectal cancer (HNPCC). The rapid progression through the adenoma/dysplasia phase occurs because of already-existing genetic perturbations, with the result of predominantly right-sided lesions.*

increased risk in those who are rapid acetylators.[22] Heterocyclic amines are formed by high-temperature cooking of meat (red or white) and fish, especially when exposed to direct flame. These heterocyclic amines may undergo oxidation and/or acetylation and eventually be converted into carcinogens that are known to induce colorectal cancer in rodents and alter DNA bases, thus inducing mutations. Oxidation, in the liver, and acetylation are under control of genetically determined enzymes. Cooking methodologies may well be critically important to the risk status in fast acetylators.[23]

Mechanisms by which genes are damaged[3]
Point mutation

Point mutation (i.e. a change in a single base pair) affects a range of genes important in human colorectal tumorigenesis. These include *ras*, *APC*, and *p53*. Carcinogens and inflammation act to cause mutations in this way. Inflammation gives rise to reactive oxygen species, which create several forms of DNA damage, including point mutations and strand breaks.

DNA rearrangement

Gene expression can also be modified by gross rearrangement of DNA sequences. Chronic myelogenous leukemia is the classic example. With progression during tumorigenesis in the colon, chromosomal breaks and rearrangements become progressively frequent due to genomic instability, and so change the function of genes that maintain normal cell behavior.

DNA deletion

Genes that maintain normal cellular homeostasis, especially proliferation and apoptosis, are known as tumor suppressor genes. Unlike oncogenes, which exert their influence by becoming active, these genes play a role because they are inactivated. Although a cell carries two copies of a gene as insurance against this, either inheritance of one defective allele or acquisition of genomic instability during tumorigenesis increases the risk due to inactivation of the other. As a consequence, loss of DNA is a major mechanism for inactivation of tumor suppressor genes.

Inactivation of DNA repair

When DNA is damaged (e.g. by carcinogens), it is repaired by specific proteins that excise the damaged DNA and repair the defect by matching it against the complementary DNA strand.[19] Of significance in the gastrointestinal tract is inactivation of the mismatch-repair (MMR) system for DNA (Figure 3.9), since this is responsible for ensuring accurate copying of DNA during cell replication. Germline mutations in *hMSH2*, *hMLH1*, *hPMS2*, *hPMS1*, and *hMSH6* – genes that encode the repair proteins – have been identified and shown to be the major causes of HNPCC (see Chapter 6). Somatic inactivation of these MMR genes has also been identified in sporadic tumors. Defective MMR means that point mutations may more easily transmit during cell replication.

DNA amplification and altered methylation of DNA are additional mechanisms by which gene expression becomes disordered in tumorigenesis.

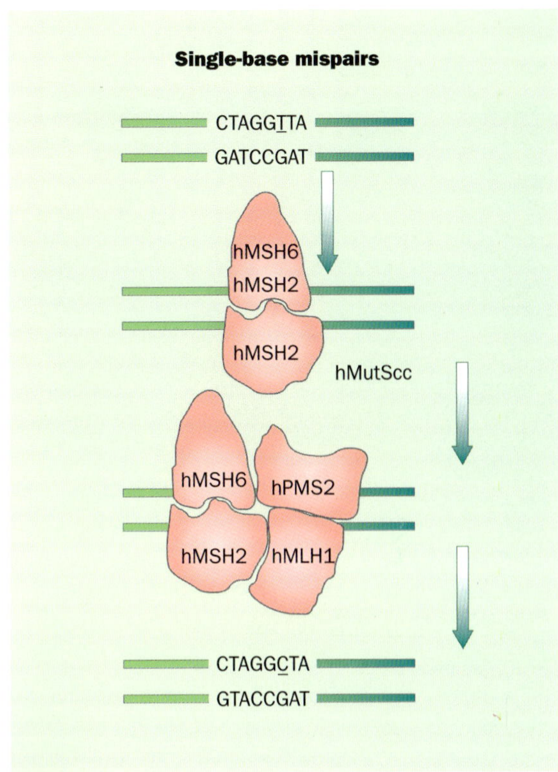

Figure 3.9 *Example of DNA mismatch repair. Mismatch-repair proteins identify mistakes after DNA replication and set up the repair. The mistake is excised and correct bases inserted. In this example, the incorrect base thymidine (T) is replaced by the correct base cytosine (C). Adapted from reference 3, with permission from the publishers Lippincott Williams and Wilkins.*

Biological impotance of genetic events

Key genes, their function, and their mechanism of alteration are listed in Table 3.2.

Important specific genes
The APC (adenomatous polyposis coli) gene – the gatekeeper for adenomas

FAP is due to an inherited mutation in the tumor suppressor gene *APC*. *APC* is the gatekeeper for adenoma formation in FAP.[6] Nonsense mutations of the *APC* gene lead to a shortened (truncated) and dysfunctional protein, with resultant defective regulation of cell death due to loss of its function. It is thought that the defective protein from the mutated allele may interfere with the normal function of the normal protein from the normal allele in some instances, but many adenomas show a loss of the second normal allele due to DNA loss resulting from deletion or rearrangement.

Table 3.2 *Major genes that may be abnormal in colorectal cancer, and their function*

Gene	Chromosomal location	Function
Tumor suppressor genes		
p53	17p	Initiates apoptosis in response to DNA damage
APC	5q	Regulates binding of β-catenin
MSH2	2p	DNA mismatch repair
MLH1	3p	DNA mismatch repair
PMS1	2q	DNA mismatch repair
PMS2	7p	DNA mismatch repair
MLH6	2p	DNA mismatch repair
p16	9p	Inhibits CDK4 and CDK6 and so controls cell cycle
SMAD4	18q	TGF-β signal transduction
DCC	18q	Netrin-1 receptor
Oncogenes		
K-ras		Membrane-associated ATPase
myc		DNA-binding protein and hence transcription regulation
myb		DNA-binding protein and hence transcription regulation

ras gene mutations

For a small adenoma to progress, additional changes must occur. In adenomas, mutations have been identified in the K-ras proto-oncogene.[15] Mutations at certain critical positions in the gene alter the Ras protein such that extracellular signaling of proliferation is constitutively activated, thus causing a gain in function even when the other allele is normal. Such mutations are seen in many colorectal neoplasms.

The p53 gene – gatekeeper for progression to cancer

Advanced adenomas remain benign while they have not invaded the muscularis mucosae. A gene often associated with malignant conversion is the p53 gene, which is affected by the two-hit mechanism characteristic of tumor suppressor genes.[18] A mutation in one allele must be associated with loss of the other allele for function to be compromised. p53 normally prevents cell replication after damage to DNA. Inactivation of the gene permits mutated DNA to be passed on to cell progeny. Mutations in p53 are usually missense in that they lead to a stable and over-expressed but non-functional p53 protein.

Other genetic alterations in colorectal cancer

Other genetic abnormalities occur in colorectal neoplasia, and may participate in multistep carcinogenesis. For example: amplification of the myc oncogene, hypomethylation of DNA, and activation of the cellular proto-oncogene src. Other oncogenes are mutated or otherwise abnormally regulated in colorectal cancer, but their roles in car-cinogenesis remain to be elucidated. Cyclooxygenase-2 is often overexpressed in colorectal cancers – this is associated with disordered apoptosis and resistance to chemotherapeutic drugs.

Genomic instability in colorectal cancer

The critical caretaker function lost in colorectal tumorigenesis is the destabilization of DNA replication, resulting in genomic instability.[1,3] This accelerates the accumulation of genetic abnormalities throughout the genome. Even though many will not be relevant to the neoplastic process, an occasional rare event will occur that alters biology, allowing a cell and its progeny to overgrow its neighbors. There are two types of genomic instability: chromosomal instability with loss of heterozygosity, and microsatellite instability.

Chromosomal instability

This type of genomic instability is found in most colorectal cancers, and results from asymmetric division of chromosomes during mitosis such that one progeny gets both copies of a gene while the other gets neither. This problem is characterized by aneuploidy, i.e. an abnormal complement of DNA, and loss of heterozygosity (LOH), i.e. loss of the two copies of a gene. By chance, LOH may result in the loss of copies of tumor suppressor genes.

Microsatellite instability

A second genetic pathway for colorectal tumorigenesis has emerged during the search for the genetic disorder responsible for HNPCC. Repetitive segments of DNA between coding areas, called microsatellites, were found to be highly susceptible to mutation in HNPCC tumors. Mutations in these are termed microsatellite instability (often termed MSI). This reflects sensitivity to mutation resulting from defects in the repair of DNA. While characteristic of HNPCC, microsatellite instability is also found in about 15–20% of sporadic, non-familial colorectal cancers, particularly those in the proximal colon. Neoplasms with microsatellite instability did not demonstrate the chaotic nuclear disorganization produced by LOH, and are more likely to be diploid than aneuploid.

Genetic pathways of colorectal tumorigenesis

The generalized pathway for tumorigenesis shown in Figure 3.6 represents on overview of the most common genetic abnormalities associated with many colorectal cancers, especially sporadic (sometimes called common) colorectal cancer. A range of observations suggest that the adenoma phase is about 5 years while the cancer phase is also up to 5 years in duration (Figure 3.5).[12,13]

Other pathways appear to exist, which vary in biological and/or genetic sequence and speed of progression (Table 3.3).

In FAP, a similar pattern of genetic changes is seen, but the ubiquitous presence of *APC* mutations in all colonic epithelial cells leads to a much earlier formation of massive numbers of adenomas.

In HNPCC, the process is quite different. Carcinomas arise rapidly through small precursor polypoid and flat adenomas owing to an accumulation of oncogene mutations or suppressor gene deletions. Tumor pathology also differs: more mucinous tumors at a more proximal location and a more prominent lymphoid reaction. Microsatellite instability due to defective DNA mismatch repair is the hallmark feature of this pathway, which does not usually involve *APC*, K-*ras*, or *p53*, but commonly involves abnormalities in TGF-β.

In colorectal carcinoma complicating longstanding ulcerative colitis, there is no precursor polyp, and the cancer develops from a dysplastic focus that may assume a raised plaque-like appearance. The molecular pathway is not well defined, but *p53* mutations occur early in dysplasia, which is different from the sequence seen in sporadic cancer.

At present, the possibility of even another molecular pathway for the 'de novo' cancers observed especially in Japan remains to be explored.

External regulation of colorectal tumorigenesis

The wide variation in international incidences of colorectal cancer suggests the importance of external regulatory factors.[2] In addition, ethnic groups migrating from low-risk into high-risk regions quite rapidly experience an increase in the incidence of colorectal cancer. Epidemiological studies looking for environmental associations with such phenomena have found that a large proportion of this variance is related to the dietary lifestyle itself. As is apparent from the discussion above on the process of tumorigenesis and the mechanisms of genomic change that lead to cancers, much of these must be acquired. However, dietary factors do more than influence changes in DNA – they also, and perhaps at least as importantly, regulate the biological consequences of altered DNA. First, we shall discuss the common aspects by which diet might regulate tumorigenesis, and then outline the mechanisms possibly operative for certain nutrients.

Table 3.3 *Alternative molecular pathways for colorectal cancer and characteristics of the process and the cancers*

Type	Characteristics			
	Relative speed of progression	**Adenomas**	**Age for cancer appearance**	**Colon cancer site**
Sporadic	Slow	Few	>50 years	Distal
FAP	Moderate	Polyposis	>15 years	Distal
HNPCC	Rapid	Relatively few	>30 years	Proximal
Ulcerative colitis	Uncertain	Flat dysplasia	Varies	Varies
"De novo"	Uncertain	Flat dysplasia	Varies	Uncertain

General themes explaining dietary regulation

Many possible general themes account for external regulation of tumorigenesis (Table 3.4). The luminal environment within the colon seems likely to play a major role as it is subject to great variation related to diet,[24] but systemic and epithelial factors are of relevance as well.

Luminal factors

The luminal environment is complex and subject to great variation. Apart from unabsorbed dietary factors, whether or not modified by digestion, the influence of luminal bacteria and their metabolic activity seem likely to be important. Furthermore, diet (including fluid intake) influences transit rates and determines fecal bulk. Hastened transit may serve to reduce exposure times to dietary carcinogens, and increased bulk may dilute them. Dietary fiber has been shown to bind and inactivate luminal carcinogens as well.[1]

Bacteria ferment unabsorbed carbohydrate (non-starch polysaccharides and starch resistant to digestion) to produce the short-chain fatty acids acetic, propionic, and butyric. This acidifies the luminal environment, and an acid environment seems to be associated with a lower risk for colorectal cancer. Butyrate has a broad range of biological actions of relevance to suppression of tumorigenesis, including an ability to promote cell maturity and facilitate apoptosis.[25] In the test tube, it directly regulates certain genes of importance in tumor development. There is increasing evidence, though yet incomplete, that different bacterial species (probiotics) are associated with a healthier luminal environment. Whether we eventually confirm that probiotics, commonly taken as yoghurt, are beneficial, remains to be seen. The observations that bacteria can also activate or inactivate carcinogens, modify bile salts to more toxic forms, and generate differential amounts of short-chain fatty acids, suggests that they may significantly influence tumorigenesis.

Endogenous luminal factors may also play a role. Bile salt composition and amount are altered by changes in pH and dietary fats.[26] Different types of fatty diet are associated with different rates of tumorigenesis. It has been suggested that secondary bile salts such as deoxycholic and lithocholic acids, produced by bacterial action in the colonic lumen, act as tumor promoters or indeed carcinogens. They are toxic to the epithelium and stimulate proliferation.

Epithelial factors

In the skin, the rate of cell proliferation at the time of exposure to a carcinogen has a major impact, because DNA is more sensitive to carcinogens during the S phase (time of DNA synthesis) of the cell cycle. Such an idea has been proposed for the colon, but has never been substantiated because of conflicting observations. It is well known that dietary fiber, especially when actively fermented in the colon, stimulates epithelial proliferation and maintains epithelial cell mass, thus preventing atrophy and maintaining integrity of the epithelial barrier.[27] Overall, fiber is protective against colorectal tumorigenesis. On the other hand, toxic bile salts seem to promote tumorigenesis and certainly stimulate epithelial proliferation, which could be a step to carcinogenesis.

Certain procarcinogens require activation to become carcinogenic. The compounds generated by high-temperature cooking of animal protein, such as PhIP (a phenylimidazopyridine) and IQ (an imidazoquinoline), fall into this category and their activation depends on the genetic polymorphisms associated with acetylator status. Those who inherit a fast-acetylator status may be more at risk of colorectal tumorigenesis,[23] especially if they eat large

Table 3.4 *Factors that may regulate colorectal tumorigenesis, classified by site of action*

Site	Examples	Risk/preventive factors
Luminal	Bacteria Transit rate Bulk and dilution Bile salt type and modification pH	Short-chain fatty acids Long-chain fatty acids Calcium Carcinogens Dietary fiber intake
Epithelial	Rate of proliferation Procarcinogen activation Phytochemicals	Permeability Apoptosis threshold
Systemic	Fish oil Physical inactivity	Non-steroidal anti-inflammatory drugs Body mass index > 30

quantities of heavily cooked meat (red or otherwise, including fish), because there is activation of these pro-carcinogens in epithelial mitochondria. Whether there are other such examples remains to be determined.

Programmed cell death or apoptosis, as outlined above, becomes progressively disordered in colorectal tumorigenesis, in part as a result of the genetic aberrations that accumulate. Certain diet-derived agents or dietary components facilitate apoptosis by altering the cellular threshold for its activation.[25] These include curcumin in curry, omega-3 fatty acids in fish oil, and butyrate from fermentation of polysaccharides. The biological concept is that activation of apoptosis leads to more efficient removal of cells with damaged DNA. Experimental studies suggest it to be of importance, but there is a lack of definitive proof establishing it as the fundamental way in which dietary factors regulate tumorigenesis by directly influencing epithelial behavior.

Systemic factors

The relevance of diet-dependent systemic factors is less obvious for colorectal tumorigenesis than the above three mechanisms, but still seems to be important. For instance, dietary fish oil seems to be protective.[28] This may be via its effects on mucosal prostaglandin production and on membrane lipid composition. Both are influenced in the colon after absorption of the lipids in the small intestine. Certainly, non-steroidal anti-inflammatory drugs have a systemic action on tumorigenesis, and perhaps achieve this by regulating apoptosis.[29]

Specific dietary components and tumorigenesis

A report from the World Cancer Research Fund has examined in depth the relationships between diet and colorectal cancer[2] and discusses the possible mechanisms. The following discussion touches on the mechanisms of a few of these relevant foods. See Table 3.5.

Dietary fats

The mechanism by which a diet rich in fats enhances tumorigenesis relates in part to their effect on bile acids and subsequent effect on colonic epithelial proliferation. Increasing animal fat intake increases total fecal bile acid and fatty acid excretion in humans. Experimental models show increased cellular proliferation and increased reactive oxygen radicals in the colon of animals on a high-fat diet.

Other oils, however, seem protective. Fish oils are rich in omega-3 polyunsaturated fatty acids, and geographical regions where people consume large amounts of fish tend to have lower incidences of colorectal cancer. Fish oils protect against colorectal cancer in animal models. The mechanism by which they protect remains uncertain, but reduction of mucosal prostaglandins in colorectal tumors may be part of the explanation.

Non-digestible polysaccharides, including dietary fiber

Dietary fiber consists of a heterogeneous mixture of non-starch polysaccharides, undigested starch (resistant starch), and other plant-derived products such as lignin. A

Table 3.5 *Examples of dietary factors that regulate tumorigenesis and how they may achieve this*

Food	Mechanism	Risk for cancer
Saturated fats, *n*-6 polyunsaturated fats	Increased bile salts, increase epithelial proliferation, increase oxygen free radicals	Increased
Fish oil	Decreases prostaglandins	Decreased
Fiber and resistant starch	Increase bulk, transit rate, and short-chain fatty acid concentrations. Bind carcinogens, alter bacterial species, decrease pH.	Decreased
Meat (red and white, excluding fish)	Possibly undigested protein is fermented to form toxic compounds	Increased
Charred meats	Increased procarcinogens	Increased
Calcium	Precipitates free fatty acids and decreases damage	Decreased
Phytochemicals	Detoxify toxins, induce metabolizing enzymes, antioxidants	Decreased

number of mechanisms seem likely to explain their protective action against colorectal cancer. Fiber hastens luminal transit time and, together with water, increases fecal bulk as a result of fermentation, thus tending to dilute the concentration of other luminal constituents.[1] Both of these would minimize contact between carcinogens and colonic epithelium. Fiber polymers can bind toxic substances and prevent them from making contact with epithelium. As outlined above, they are also subject to fermentation by luminal anaerobic flora, which reduces fecal pH and generates short-chain fatty acids. One of these, butyric acid, is present in high concentrations in the colonic lumen and is an important energy source for colonic epithelium.[25] Different fiber sources vary in their capacities to alter these factors, but all mechanisms seem likely to be important to varying degrees. The strongest support for a protective role comes from early experiments using wheat bran.[30]

Dietary protein

There is a strong association between colorectal cancer and red meat consumption above 80–140 g per day.[31] The mechanism for this is unclear, and appears to be independent of fat content. Undigested protein is fermented by colonic bacteria to produce a range of toxic nitrogenous compounds; this, plus the iron content and means of cooking, have all been suggested as being responsible.

Micronutrients

Micronutrients are specific chemicals in the diet that do not supply energy but are nutritionally relevant. Our understanding of how these interact with the process of tumorigenesis is developing. What follows is a short summary of some of the relevant or topical issues from a mechanistic perspective. The reader is directed to reference 2 for supporting detail.

Calcium Calcium tends to normalize the generalized disturbance in the regulation of cell proliferation seen in the colons of patients with adenomatous polyps or cancers. It has been suggested that luminal calcium could reduce the damaging and mitogenic effects of free fatty acids and bile acids by precipitating free fatty acids as calcium soaps.

Selenium Reduced levels of selenium have been associated with an increased risk for colorectal cancer, and some view it as an antioxidant. It is a constituent of the enzyme glutathione peroxidase, which prevents damage to tissue by free radicals; it also minimizes toxicity caused by certain heavy metals.

Vitamins A, C, and E Indirect studies show that these agents have promise as anticarcinogens, especially because of their powerful antioxidant activities. Retinoids also function as differentiating agents and reduce epithelial proliferation. The impact of these agents has not been obvious in interventional studies, and this suggests that antioxidant activities are not sufficiently powerful to suppress tumorigenesis in the colon. It seems that other substances in the food sources of these agents also are contributing to the protective actions.

Folate Folate status relates to risk for cancer. Folate-replete animals are less susceptible to tumorigenesis since they are less at risk of DNA hypomethylation, a nonspecific effect on DNA that can result in changes in gene regulation.

Other phytochemicals A range of other components in plant foods, especially those strongly associated with protection and found in fresh vegetables, are summarized in Chapters 4 and 5. Their mechanisms of action include inactivation of carcinogens, detoxification, and scavenging of free radicals. They include benzyl isothiocyanate, a naturally occurring constituent of cruciferous vegetables, organosulfur compounds from *Allium* species (i.e. the garlic and onion families), monoterpenes found in citrus fruits, polyphenols in teas, flavones, tannins, protease inhibitors, terpenes, curcumin, glycerrhetinic acid, and glucarates. Many of these agents have been proposed as potential chemopreventive substances for human studies.

Carcinogens and procarcinogens in foods

From the perspective of colorectal cancer, there are no known naturally occurring colorectal carcinogens in food. However, carcinogens may be produced during cooking of meats as described above or may be derived from endogenous bile salts subjected to metabolic changes by colonic bacteria.

Conclusions

Colorectal cancer is a genetic disorder in which most of the genetic abnormalities are acquired but some are inherited. Colorectal cancer develops by a process termed 'multistep carcinogenesis', driven by mutations and other genetic abnormalities, randomly occurring at different points in time, at multiple sites on DNA. The whole process may take as long as 10 years but it can be accelerated in certain familial cancer settings. Benign dysplasia precedes invasive cancer, the former often taking the form of an adenomatous polyp. The principal types of genetic disorders are an unstable genome and abnormalities in particular genes. Of the latter, tumor suppressor genes and oncogenes are those most often involved. Some of these genetic disorders and the resultant biological disturbances can be regulated by dietary lifestyle. There are a variety of mechanisms responsible for such regulation, but many act via changes in the colonic luminal environment. Better understanding of the process of colorectal tumorigenesis thus enables us to devise better ways to slow or block the process and so prevent this cancer causing death and morbidity.

References (*Reviews and general articles)

1. *Boland CR, Malignant tumors of the colon. In: *Textbook of Gastroenterology*, 3rd edn (Yamada T, Alpers DH, Laine L et al, eds). Philadelphia: Lippincott, Williams & Wilkins, 1999:2023–82.

2. *World Cancer Research Fund and American Institute for Cancer Research, *Food, Nutrition and the Prevention of Cancer; A Global Perspective*. Washington, DC: American Institute for Cancer Research, 1997.

3. *Carethers JM, Boland CR, Neoplasia of the gastrointestinal tract. In: *Textbook of Gastroenterology*, 3rd edn (Yamada T, Alpers DH, Laine L et al, eds). Philadelphia Lippincott, Williams & Wilkins, 1999: 585–610.

4. Carson DA, Ribeiro JM, Apoptosis and disease. *Lancet* 1993; **341:** 1251–4.

5. Morin PJ, Vogelstein B, Kinzler KW, Apoptosis and APC in colorectal tumorigenesis. *Proc Natl Acad Sci USA* 1996; **93:** 7950–4.

6. Aberle H, Schwartz H, Kemler R, Cadherin-catenin complex: protein interactions and their implications for cadherin function. *J Cell Biochem* 1996; **61:** 514–23.

7. Kinzler K, Vogelstein B, Gatekeepers and caretakers. *Nature* 1997; **386:** 761–3.

8. *Fearon ER, Vogelstein B, A genetic model for colorectal tumorigenesis. *Cell* 1990; **61:** 759–67.

9. *Morson BC, Evolution of cancer of colon and rectum. *Cancer* 1974; **34:** 845–9.

10. Muto T, Bussey HJR, Morson BC, The evolution of cancer of the colon and rectum. *Cancer* 1975; **36:** 2251–70.

11. *Atkin WS, Morson BC, Cuzick J, Long-term risk of colorectal cancer after excision of rectosigmoid adenomas. *N Engl J Med* 1992; **326:** 658–62.

12. Kozuka S, Nogaki M, Ozeki T et al, Premalignancy of the mucosal polyp in the large intestine. II. Estimation of the periods required for malignant transformation of mucosal polyps. *Dis Colon Rectum* 1975; **18:** 494–500.

13. *Winawer SJ, Zauber AG, Ho MN et al, Prevention of colorectal cancer by colonoscopic polypectomy. *N Engl J Med* 1993; **329:** 1977–81.

14. Kuramoto S, Oohara T, Minute cancers arising de novo in the human large intestine. *Cancer* 1988; **61:** 829–34.

15. *Vogelstein B, Fearon ER, Hamilton SR et al, Genetic alterations during colorectal-tumor development. *N Engl J Med* 1988; **319:** 525–32.

16. Powell SM, Zilz N, Beazer-Barclay Y et al, *APC* mutations occur early during colorectal tumorigenesis. *Nature* 1992; **359:** 235–7.

17. Law DJ, Olschwang S, Monpezat J-P et al, Concerted nonsyntenic allelic loss in human colorectal carcinoma. *Science* 1988; **241:** 961–5.

18. Kikuchi-Yanoshita R, Konishi M, Ito S et al, Genetic changes of both P53 alleles associated with the conversion from colorectal adenoma to early carcinoma in familial adenomatous polyposis and non-familial adenomatous polyposis patients. *Cancer Res* 1992; **52:** 3965–71.

19. Lengauer C, Kinzler KW, Vogelstein B, Genetic instability in colorectal cancers. *Nature* 1997; **386:** 623–7.

20. Lang NP, Butler MA, Massergill J et al, Rapid metabolic phenotypes for acetyltransferase and cytochrome p4501A2 and putative exposure to food-borne heterocyclic amines increase the risk for colorectal cancer or polyps. *Cancer Epidemiol Biomarkers Prev* 1994; **3:** 675–82.

21. Miller EC, Miller JA, Searches for ultimate chemical carcinogens and their reactions with cellular macromolecules. *Cancer* 1981; **47:** 2327–45.

22. Loeb LA, Mutator phenotype may be required for multistage carcinogenesis. *Cancer Res* 1991; **51:** 3075–9.

23. Roberts-Thomson IC, Ryan P, Khoo KK et al, Diet, acetylator phenotype and risk of colorectal neoplasia. *Lancet* 1996; **347:** 1372–4.

24. *Cummings JH, Wiggins HS, Jenkins DJA et al, Influence of diets high and low in animal fat on bowel habit, gastro-intestinal transit, fecal microflora, bile acid and fat excretion. *J Clin Invest* 1978; **61:** 953–63.

25. *Young GP, Gibson PR, Butyrate and the human cancer cell. In: *Physiological and Clinical Aspects of Short Chain Fatty Acid Metabolism* (Cummings J, Sakata T, Rombeau JL eds). Cambridge: Cambridge University Press, 1994: 319–35.

26. Reddy BS, Dietary fat and its relationship to large bowel cancer. *Cancer Res* 1981; **41:** 3700–5.

27. Cummings JH, Cellulose and the human gut, *Gut* 1984; **25:** 805–10.

28. Anti M, Marra G, Armelao F et al, Effect of ω-3 fatty acids on rectal mucosal cell proliferation in subjects at risk for colon cancer. *Gastroenterology* 1992; **103:** 883–91.

29. Piazza GA, Kulchak Rahm AL, Krutzsch M et al, Antineoplastic drugs sulindac sulfide and sulfone inhibit cell growth in inducing apoptosis. *Cancer Res* 1995; **55:** 3110–6.

30. MacLennan R, Macrae F, Ward M et al, Randomized trial of intake of fat, fiber and betacarotene to prevent colorectal adenomas. *J Natl Cancer Inst* 1995; **87:** 1760–6.

31. Giovannucci E, Rimm EB, Stampfer MJ et al, Intake of fat, meat, and fiber in relation to risk of colon cancer in men. *Cancer Res* 1994; **54:** 2390–7.

4 Is diet important in preventing colorectal cancer?

Paul Rozen, Bernard Levin, Graeme P Young

Introduction

From studies of migrants moving from areas of low colorectal cancer incidence to westernized countries having a high incidence, it became apparent that within one or two generations, these immigrants developed cancer rates similar to those of the indigenous populations of the host countries. This pointed to the environment as providing the main risk factors for colorectal neoplasia, the most logical conclusions being that diet and lifestyle are the main etiologies in at least 30% of the cases. This does not negate the importance of genetic risk factors in dominant high-penetrance disorders such as familial adenomatous polyposis, hereditary non-polyposis colorectal cancer, or chronic and extensive inflammatory bowel disease. However, these can only contribute to about 3–5% of colorectal cancer cases. The remainder are probably explained by the widespread presence of inherited low-penetrance genetic perturbations that interact with environmental factors and lead to adenoma and/or cancer of the large bowel.[1,2] So, even though diet has a very important role in the etiology of large-bowel cancer, we must also take into consideration interaction with race, gender, genetic make-up, and lifestyle.[3] These are discussed in Chapter 2.

What preventive dietary recommendations can we make?

What is the relevance of body weight?

A higher than recommended body weight is a preventable risk factor for important chronic disorders such as cardiovascular disease, and several common cancers such as the hormone-dependent malignancies and colorectal cancer or adenomas.[4–8] It is well known from both experimental studies in animals and from human epidemiological studies that the risk for colorectal neoplasia, adenomas, or cancer, is related to the caloric intake and *body mass index* (BMI).[6] This is illustrated by the observation that it is easier to promote cancer in the overweight experimental animal than in the active, non-obese rodent.[9] In humans, the risk for neo-plasia, including that of the large bowel, is statistically most significant in the extreme of obesity. Measurement of body weight is scientifically less useful than the BMI, which takes into account both weight and height, the formula being weight in kilograms divided by height in square centimeters (W/H^2).[6] A simplified classification of weight status and risk for colorectal cancer is given in Table 4.1.

Calories

In practice, the first consideration is the *total amount of calories* that we eat. Clearly, the amount ingested should depend on what we need to replace our daily expenditure. In a westernized society, once we grow to adulthood and become physically less active, we tend to continue with previous dietary habits and not reduce our caloric intake in line with reduced needs. So, in general, being mildly to moderately overweight is a common phenomenon in men, and is also a problem in the economically disadvantaged of both sexes due to the easier availability of cheap but high-calorie foods. Another recent phenomenon is the overfeeding of these same foods to infants, so it is not uncommon to see overweight babies and children. Maintaining close-to-ideal body weight is a lifetime habit, and should be instilled by parents from childhood.

Table 4.1 *Body Mass Index (BMI),[a] approximate classification of weight status, and risk for colorectal and other cancers*

		Cancer risk[b]	
BMI range	**Weight status**	**Any**	**Colorectal**
10–<18.5	Underweight		
18.5–<25	Ideal weight		
25–<30	Overweight		
30–<40	Obese	Yes	
40–70	Gross obesity		Yes

[a] BMI = weight in kg/height in cm².
[b] Derived from references 1, 4, and 6.

Are there commonly consumed dietary additives or contaminants that have been identified as certain carcinogens?

Considerable public health efforts have and are being made to maintain the optimal quality of water and food products. This has included the identification and removal from consumption of those substances that are potentially carcinogenic, such as the breakdown products of fertilizers, preservatives, food colors, and antibacterial or antifungal agents (none of which are known to cause colorectal neoplasia). In westernized countries, this goal has been achieved; known carcinogens are searched for and contaminated foods destroyed before marketing.[3,10] Chlorinated water has been extensively investigated, and has not been proven to be a risk factor for colon cancer.[4]

What should we eat so as to minimize the risk for colorectal cancer?

In contrast to the experimental animal, which is constantly fed a diet whose constituents have been artificially standardized, the free-living human eats a mixed diet. This diet varies from day to day, by seasons, changing tastes, and habits, and with age. So, it is difficult to draw conclusions for humans from animal studies and from the epidemiological studies of populations that are not uniform genetically, or by gender, or in their diet and lifestyle habits.[4,5]

Almost all the constituents of our usual diet have been identified both by epidemiologists and from experimental studies to have some measure of cancer-promoting or cancer-preventive value (Table 4.2). However, in general, these have only a mild to moderate influence on the process of carcinogenesis, especially when contrasting the occasional intake of a specific food within a mixed diet to the constant habit of tobacco smoking. Even so, the following conclusions can be drawn regarding food constituents and specific foods. Their use as short-term dietary supplements is also described in Chapter 5.

Main food constituents ('macronutrients')

Fats

The evidence of a strong relationship between the amount of fat ingested and the risk for large-bowel neoplasia is less clear in humans than from animal studies, where induction of tumors is easier when the dietary intake of fat is increased. In the US population, dietary fat of animal origin is regarded as an important risk factor for colorectal cancer, especially when taking into account the major contribution that dietary fat makes to the total caloric intake, and as a means of cooking.[4,10] But, in European and Mediterranean populations, the evidence is less conclusive, since there are countries, such as Greece, southern Italy, and Spain, where there is a relatively high intake of different types of fat and yet the incidence of large-bowel cancer is not high.[4] These countries have a high intake of fish, whose oil contains omega-3 fatty acids, and olive oil containing monounsaturated fat, which seem neutral or protective, while the animal fats in the US diet may be more of a risk factor.[11,12]

There has been a strong recommendation in the USA to reduce total fat intake to 30–35% of total caloric intake, and this seems to have contributed to the marked reduction that recently occurred in the incidence of coronary artery disease. It is still not clear if this is the reason for the slight reduction in the incidence of large-bowel cancer that has recently occurred in the American Caucasian female population, but not in males (see Chapter 2).

Carbohydrates

Studies of animal models of carcinogenesis and some epidemiological studies of large-bowel neoplasia both showed an inverse relationship between increased total carbohydrate intake and risk for colorectal adenomas.[4,7] The strongest evidence for protection is from ingestion of complex, long-chain carbohydrates, rather than from the simple sugar sucrose. Actually, in some studies, both experimental and epidemiological, a high intake of sucrose was found to potentiate the risk for colorectal cancer.[4] A consistently high intake of sucrose is probably accompanied by a relatively low intake of other dietary constituents, including protective dietary factors. It has also been suggested that persistent hyperglycemia, and consequent insulin response, is a stimulus for colonic epithelial proliferation and risk for cancer.[8] The complex-carbohydrate-containing foods should provide 45–60% of the total energy intake and refined sugar less than 10%.[4]

Fiber and fluid intake

The fermentation breakdown products of complex carbohydrates are important in maintaining healthy colonic epithelial cells and bowel function. In addition, meta-analysis of epidemiological studies evaluating fiber intake in preventing colorectal cancer indicates a low but protective role for fiber, especially from that of wheat origin.[4,7,10,13–15] However, this protection could not be confirmed in a recent analysis examining the long-term intake of relatively low amounts of dietary fiber by nurses and their risk for large-bowel cancer, or by other prospective studies.[15,16] Additionally, various interven-

Table 4.2 Lifestyle and dietary factors and their estimated relative roles in colorectal carcinogenesis

Lifestyle/dietary factor	Relative role	Protective	Promoting
Physical activity	Moderate	+	
Total caloric intake	Moderate		+
Obesity	Minor		+
Alcohol	Minor		+
Tobacco	Minor		+
Chronic NSAID[a] use	Moderate	+	
Total fluid intake	Minor	+	
Tea	Minor	+	
Fried, charred, smoked foods	Moderate		+
Total fat intake	Major		+
Animal fat	Moderate		+
Fish oil	Minor	+	
Olive oil	Minor	+	
Total carbohydrate intake	Moderate	+	
Wheat bran	Moderate	+	
Cane sugar	Minor		+
Micronutrients	Moderate	+	
Calcium	Minor	+	
Iron	Minor		+
Beef	Moderate		+
Poultry	Minor	+	
Vegetables	Minor	+	
Fruits	Minor	+	
Milk products (low fat)	Minor	+	

[a]Non-steroidal anti-inflammatory drug.

tion trials with dietary fiber supplements did not demonstrate a marked effect on reducing adenoma recurrence.[4]

It was recently shown in epidemiological studies of both colorectal cancer and adenoma patients that the protective effect provided by fiber was potentiated by the individual's total fluid intake. The type and source of fiber ingested, and types and amounts of other dietary constituents (e.g. fat, calcium, and fluid), are likely to influence the protective role that fiber has to play within the intracolonic environment.[7,15] The recommended daily intake of fiber is 25–35 g.[4,15]

Protein

As protein is derived from both vegetable and animal sources, it is difficult to evaluate its role in colorectal carcinogenesis separately from these food sources or from the means of food preparation. There is a little evidence relating protein intake per se to neoplasia; the protein foods and the effects of their cooking are discussed below.[4]

Minor dietary constituents ('micronutrients')

These are the vitamins and minerals that have been extensively investigated and, in the main, are protective against colorectal cancer. Their anticarcinogenic roles seem to be minor, acting on the intraluminal contents and/or by strengthening of the resistance of the large-bowel epithelium to carcinogens. The list of these nutrients is long and they have various functions; they include selenium, calcium, and vitamins A (carotenoids), C, D, E, and folic acid.[17] Their pharmaceutical use as chemopreventive agents is discussed in Chapter 5. Vitamin supplements are not needed when eating the recommended five portions per day of fruits and salads.

There has been considerable interest in the colon cancer protective role of *calcium*. The strongest evidence for this is experimental, as shown by giving a 'Western-style' diet to mice and suppressing the resulting hyperproliferative response of the colonic epithelium by adding dietary calcium.[18] The epidemiological evidence is not supportive of a strong anticarcinogenic role, but rather of a modulating, protective role within a 'carcinogenic' Western diet. In adenoma patients, suppression of rectal epithelial proliferation by long-term calcium dietary supplements is greatest when their dietary intake is high in carbohydrate, fiber, and water and low in fat, and tobacco use is also low.[19] Long-term calcium supplements in humans will slightly but significantly reduce the recurrence rate of large-bowel adenomatous polyps by 18%.[20] What seems important about the calcium intake is not its source, but rather its total intake: up to 1500–2000 mg calcium ion/day. The dietary reference intake for calcium has recently been increased to 1200 mg/day for adults aged 50 years or older.[21] This discrepancy in dosage probably reflects the difference between minimal physiological needs and pharmacological effects. Very few adults have even this minimal intake when eating their 'Western' diet. The higher intake of calcium can be obtained by providing a diet rich in calcium, such as calcium-containing low-fat milk products. This diet has been shown to be practical in volunteers, and suppresses their large-bowel epithelial proliferation.[22] However, it has not been proven to prevent neoplasia, nor are its long-term effects known. Other, non-dairy sources of dietary calcium are listed in Table 4.3.

There is now some epidemiological and experimental evidence to link a high intake of *iron* and having high body stores of iron (especially due to supplements or genetic reasons for iron overload) with an increased risk for colorectal cancer. High dietary or supplemental sources of iron lead to the formation of intraluminal free radicals, which experimentally have been associated with risk for

cancer.[4,23] If confirmed, these observations may have an important implication on the clinical practice of maintaining full body stores of iron.

Bioactive compounds

This is a general term that includes numerous chemicals found in fruits, vegetables, spices, condiments, herbs, etc. that have been proven to have anticarcinogenic properties. Some of the best known and studied are those found in green tea, tomatoes, onions, carrots, lemons, curry, and garlic. A partial list is given in Table 4.4. Even though their effects have been demonstrated experimentally, it is not clear how important is their occasional ingestion in the mixed Western diet. However, there are national groups or individuals where the consistent intake of some of these compounds (e.g. green tea and curry) may play a significant anticarcinogenic role.[24,25] The consistent ingestion of isoflavonoids and lignans found in soybean and rye cereal have been associated with a lower risk of cancer, especially breast cancer, in Asia and Scandinavia.[26,27] Their effect in preventing colorectal cancer is less well documented.[27]

Specific food sources

Most evidence for or against an anticarcinogenic property of specific food groups or foods is based on epidemiological and experimental studies. However, foods vary in their composition from season to season, from one geographical area to another, and between food product manufacturers. So, it is not always possible to extrapolate from one study to another. In addition, and most importantly, we eat a mixed and varied diet, and national and personal habits change from time to time.

Cereals

In the main, countries having national habits of a high intake of complex carbohydrates, such as whole-grain wheat, rye, and pasta, have a lower incidence of colorectal and other cancers.[4,5,13,14,28,29] This is partly due to the fact that these carbohydrates displace fats as an energy source (see Figure 4.1). The recommendation for an adult is 600–800 g /day.[4]

Vegetables and fruits

As a food group, vegetables have been associated with a reduced risk for both colorectal cancer and adenomas, with less strong evidence for fruit to have a protective effect.[4,13] Fruits and vegetables contain vitamins, minerals, and some poorly digestible fiber, which clearly may all

Table 4.3 *Dietary sources and their relative calcium content*

Cheese	Highest
Kelp	
Sardines	Moderate
Vegetable greens	
Nuts	Lower
Beans	
Tofu	
Whole milk	
Spinach	
Sesame	

The above foods have a calcium content ranging from about 1000 mg/100 g in the highest calcium-containing foods to 100–200 mg/100 g in the lowest calcium-containing food.

Table 4.4 *Classification and sources of phytochemicals*[a]

Class	Sources	Action
Allium	Garlic	Induce enzymes, detoxify
Dithiolthiones	Cruciferous vegetables	Induce enzymes, detoxify
Isothiocyanates	Spices, vegetables	Induce enzymes
d-Limonene	Citrus fruits	Induce glutathione S-transferase
Phytoestrogens	Cereals, pulses	Alter steroid hormone metabolism
Flavonoids	Tea, fruit, vegetables	Antioxidants
Polyphenols	Tea, fruit, vegetables	Detoxify, inhibit *N*-nitrosation

[a] Adapted from reference 4.

play protective roles. Considerable efforts have been made to identify other protective bioactive constituents, some of which have been discussed above.[30]

Legumes, a food group including beans and nuts, are often consumed in small amounts in the mixed diet, but are staple elements of vegetarians' diets. This food family also includes soybean, which is consumed frequently in Asia. Epidemiological studies have demonstrated a lower risk for cancer in consumers of soybean.[26,27] However, this effect is less prominent in preventing large-bowel cancer than for hormone-dependent malignancies.[27] It has not been conclusively proven that the beneficial effect of legumes arises just from their contents of phytoestrogens (lignans and isoflavonoids); it could also be from other nutrients in these foods. Surprisingly, a recently published prospective study of mortality in vegetarians did not demonstrate a reduction in their cancer mortality as compared with that in non-vegetarians.[31] The recommendation for fruits and vegetables is 400–800 g/day – about five or more servings.[4]

Meat

Beef and lamb ('red' meat) and poultry and pork need to be considered separately.

Red meat

The epidemiological studies are not conclusive, but tend to indicate a risk for colorectal cancer in persons having a high dietary intake of beef (greater than 80–140 g/day).[4,10] However, it is also necessary to take into

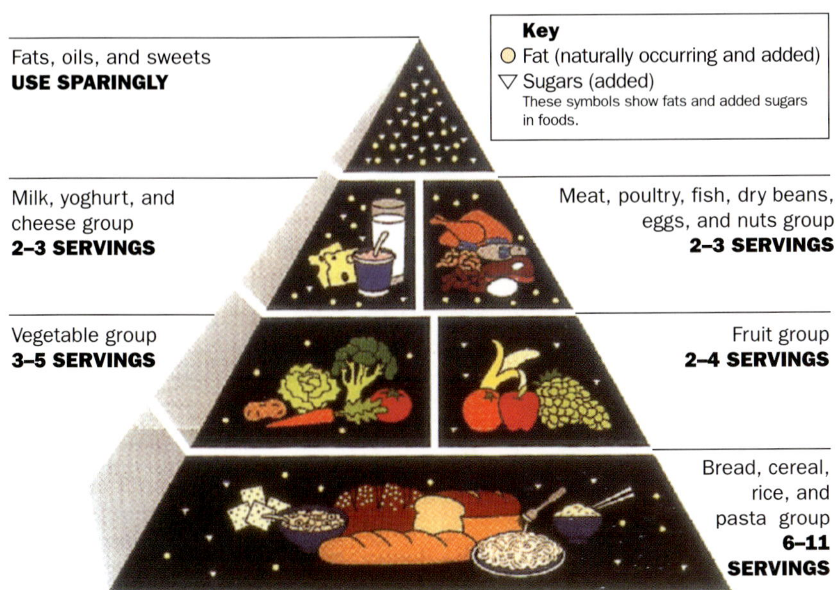

Figure 4.1 *Schematic representation of the amounts and types of food groups recommended/day to promote health. Published with permission of the Department of Agriculture, USA.*

account the meat's content of fat and iron (also from the blood), and means of cooking (e.g. fried or charred) – all of which may increase the risk for cancer.[4] Interestingly, it has recently been demonstrated that the iron-containing heme molecule from meat can result in cytotoxic and hyperproliferative effects on the colonic mucosa – more so than just mineral iron added to the diet of experimental animals.[32] The daily consumption of red meat, one adult-size serving, should be less than 80 g/day.

Poultry and pork

Here, the epidemiological evidence is that the intake of low-fat meat of poultry and pork origin is of little risk for large-bowel neoplasia.[4]

Fish

Fish from the cold-water oceans are rich in omega-3 oils, which are believed to be protective for both cardiovascular disease and colorectal neoplasia. Countries bordering the Mediterranean Sea that have a low intake of meat but a high consumption of ocean fish have less risk for large-bowel cancer.[4,5,11,12,33] This is not necessarily the case if the consumption is of pond-bred fish, since the biochemical constitution of the fish's body fat depends on its source of artificial food.

Eggs

These are obviously a rich source for fat, especially cholesterol. In the large bowel, intraluminal metabolites of cholesterol promote carcinogenesis. Eggs are probably a risk factor not only for cardiovascular disease, but also for colorectal cancer, especially in men.[4]

Milk products

These need to be considered as low- or high-fat milk products. Low-fat dairy products provide calcium and vitamin D, which may have a preventive role for large-bowel cancer – as shown by intervention studies in humans and experimental studies in animals. However, the inconsistent epidemiological evidence for a protective role for milk products might be related to the fat content of the milk and its products.[4,22]

Food preparation

The relationship of food preparation to carcinogenesis has now been extensively evaluated. High-temperature cooking by grilling, frying, and charring of meat produces heterocyclic amines, which are carcinogens.[10,34,35] Epidemiological studies of persons consistently eating such prepared

foods show that they have an increased risk for colorectal neoplasia.[4,5,36] There is evidence that this risk is greatest in persons of a specific genetic phenotype – fast acetylators – who have a reduced capability to metabolize these carcinogenic products.[37] This is further complicated by the biochemical interactions that occur during cooking between proteins and other constituents such as fats and sugars, to produce compounds that are also carcinogenic.[38]

Processing meat by smoking or curing has been associated with the production of carcinogenic nitrosamines from nitrites. Consistent intake of such products has been associated with an increased risk for large-bowel neoplasia.[4,10]

Hypothesis for colorectal carcinogenesis

Fat ingestion causes an increased flow of intestinal bile, and some of this fat and bile reach the colon, where bacteria degrade them to fatty and bile acids. These damage the large-bowel epithelium, and thus stimulate proliferation, which leaves the epithelium susceptible to carcinogenesis. The usual by-products of bile metabolism and food preparation may themselves act as carcinogens, especially if there is genetic susceptibility. In addition to these effects of foods on the intraluminal contents and bowel wall, the products of digestion are absorbed and release local peptides and hormones such as gastrin and insulin, which are also factors promoting epithelial hyperproliferation.

Dietary fiber by its bulk and fluids dilute the colonic contents and shorten transit time, permitting less time and contact of the contents with the bowel wall. The bacterial fermentation of cereal fibers produces short-chain fatty acids, which are important for the metabolism and health of the colonic epithelium, and help maintain its integrity. The resultant intraluminal acidic pH inhibits bile acid dehydroxylation and dehydrogenation, events that can lead to the production of carcinogenic by-products. Micronutrients and bioactive compounds protect through several mechanisms – systemically, they promote cell differentiation and apoptosis and help maintain epithelial integrity, while intraluminally, they help detoxify carcinogenic dietary and metabolic by-products (Figure 4.2).

Intervention trials

There have been a number of clinical trials performed, adding food items, or food groups or even modifying dietary habits.[5] Some have been completed and their results published.[4,15,33] The most important is the Women's

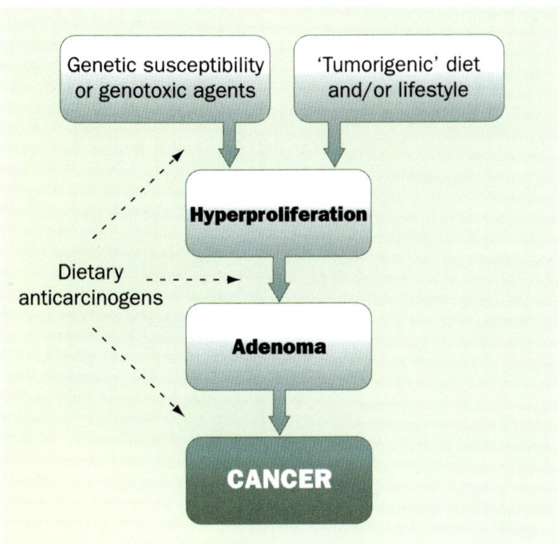

Figure 4.2 *Schematic representation of the interactions between dietary and genetic tumor-promoting factors and preventive dietary factors.*

Health Initiative, which is a very large, multifactorial trial whose results will tell us not only about the recommended relative proportions and amounts of its dietary constituents that are most health-promoting, but also about its success in modifying the dietary habits of a large healthy US population.[39] But, until there are more data, it is difficult to make recommendations other than the existing ones.

Dietary recommendations

What conclusions about diet and colorectal cancer can we draw today? Realistically, these are the same as presented a decade ago! Namely, we are dealing with an *imbalance* between protective and deleterious dietary factors and lifestyle, possibly interacting with a genetic susceptibility in some cases. There is no one individual food item or micronutrient that causes or prevents colorectal cancer, but it is the total long-term lifestyle and diet that is important (Table 4.2).

The National Academy of Sciences of the USA and the American Cancer Society feel that there is enough evidence to recommend a multipurpose 'health' regimen, good for preventing obesity, hyperlipidemia, adult-type diabetes, cardiovascular disease, and some cancers.[40]

This regimen can be summarized (and modified slightly) as follows:

1. Be physically active, eat in moderation and avoid obesity throughout life.
2. Reduce fat intake as a source of energy. Ideally, fats should not contribute more than 25–30% of daily caloric intake. Use olive or canola oils for cooking and salad dressing.
3. Substitute lean chicken, pork, fish, and low-fat dairy products for red meat.
4. Eat adequate amounts of fruits and fresh vegetables and have an adequate fluid intake.
5. Use complex carbohydrates and high-fiber grains to displace fat as an energy source.
6. Reduce alcohol consumption and cease or never begin tobacco smoking.
7. Avoid high-temperature and direct-flame overcooking of meats.

This is illustrated in Figure 4.1, which also gives an indication of the relative amounts of food types that are recommended per day. This diet and lifestyle is not only healthful, but also palatable, economical and multipurpose, for the prevention of common diseases.

Based on these recommendations, the 'Western-style' diet has been modified and is being tried in a large number (65 000) of American women.[38] Another recommended diet and lifestyle modification is that of being vegetarian. In general, studies have shown vegetarians to have less cardiovascular disease than non-vegetarians, and they were believed to have a lower mortality from cancer.[4,5] Surprisingly, this was not confirmed in a very large follow-up study of vegetarians.[31] A third dietary pattern is that of Mediterranean countries. There, a high intake of fruits, vegetables, cereals, fish and olive oil has been associated with a lower incidence of cardiovascular disease and cancer.[4,5,33]

In conclusion, the choice of any one of the above long-term diets and lifestyles is individual. Based on the numerous data available, any one of them may provide a better dietary protection against colorectal cancer than the present 'Western' diet.

References (*Reviews and general articles)

1. Lutz WK, Carcinogens in the diet vs. overnutrition. Individual dietary habits, malnutrition, and genetic susceptibility modify carcinogenic potency and cancer risk. *Mutat Res* 1999; **443**: 251–8.

2. *Manson MM, Benford DJ, Factors influencing the carcinogenicity of food chemicals. *Toxicology* 1999; **134**: 93–108.

3. Labadarios DL, Parke DV, Nutrition and diet in the prevention and treatment of cancer. *J Clin Biochem Nutr* 1999; **26**: 135–53.

4. *World Cancer Research Fund/American Institute for Cancer Research, Food, Nutrition and the Prevention of Cancer: a Global Perspective. Washington, DC: Banta Books, 1997.

5. *Schatzkin A, Dietary prevention of colorectal cancer. In: *Prevention and Early Detection of Colorectal Cancer* (Young GP, Rozen P, Levin B, eds). London: Saunders, 1996: 103–13.

6. *Ford ES, Body mass index and colon cancer in a national sample of adult US men and women. *Am J Epidemiol* 1999; **150**: 390–8.

7. *Lubin F, Rozen P, Arieli B et al, Nutritional and lifestyle habits and water-fiber interaction in colorectal adenoma etiology. *Cancer Epidemiol Biomarkers Prev* 1997; **6**: 79–85.

8. Schoen RE, Tangen CM, Kuller LH et al, Increased blood glucose and insulin, body size, and incident colorectal cancer. *J Natl Cancer Inst* 1999; **91**: 1147–54.

9. Weindruch R, Albanes D, Kritchevsky D, The role of calories and caloric restriction in carcinogenesis. *Hematol Oncol Clin North Am* 1991; **5**: 79–89.

10. Ferguson LR, Natural and man-made mutagens and carcinogens in the human diet. *Mutat Res* 1999; **443**: 1–10.

11. Rose DP, Connolly JM, Omega-3 fatty acids as cancer chemopreventive agents. *Pharmacol Ther* 1999; **83**: 217–44.

12. *de Deckere EAM, Possible beneficial effect of fish and fish *n*-3 polyunsaturated fatty acids in breast and colorectal cancer. *Eur J Cancer Prev* 1999; **8**: 213–21.

13. *Trock B, Lanza E, Greenwald P, Dietary fiber, vegetables and colon cancer: critical review and meta-analysis of the epidemiologic evidence. *J Natl Cancer Inst* 1990; **82**: 650–61.

14. *Slavin JL, Martini MC, Jacobs DR Jr et al, Plausible mechanisms for the protectiveness of whole grains. *Am J Clin Nutr* 1999; **70**(Suppl): 459S–63S.

15. *Kim Y-I, AGA technical review: impact of dietary fiber on colon cancer occurrence. *Gastroenterology* 2000; **18**: 1235–57.

16. Fuchs CS, Giovannucci EL, Colditz GA et al, Dietary fiber and the risk of colorectal cancer and adenoma in women. *N Engl J Med* 1999; **340**: 169–76.

17. *Weisburger JH, Nutritional approach to cancer prevention with emphasis on vitamins, antioxidants and carotenoids. *Am J Clin Nutr* 1991; **53**: 226S–37S.

18. Richter F, Newmark HL, Richter A et al, Inhibition of Western-diet induced hyperproliferation and hyperplasia in mouse colon by two sources of calcium. *Carcinogenesis* 1995; **16**: 2685–9.

19. Rozen P, Lubin F, Papo N et al, Calcium supplements interact significantly with long-term diet while suppressing rectal epithelial proliferation in adenoma patients. *Cancer* 2001; **91**: 833–40.

20. Baron JA, Beach M, Mandel JS et al, Calcium supplements for prevention of colorectal adenomas. *N Engl J Med* 1999; **340**: 101–7.

21. *Food and Nutrition Board, Institute of Medicine: Dietary Reference Intakes for Calcium, Phosphorus, Magnesium, Vitamin D and Fluoride.* Washington, DC: National Academy Press, 1997.

22. Holt PR, Atillasoy EO, Gilman J et al, Modulation of abnormal colonic epithelial cell proliferation and differentiation by low-fat dairy foods. *JAMA* 1998; **280**: 1074–9.

23. *Weinberg ED, The role of iron in cancer. *Eur J Cancer Prev* 1996; **5**: 19–36.

24. Ji B-T, Chow W-H, Hsing AW et al, Green tea consumption and the risk of pancreatic and colorectal cancers. *Int J Cancer* 1997; **70**: 255–8.

25. *Giovannucci E, Tomatoes, tomato-based products, lycopene, and cancer: review of the epidemiologic literature. *J Natl Cancer Inst* 1999; **91**: 317–31.

26. Thiagarajan DG, Bennink MR, Bourquin LD et al, Prevention of precancerous colonic lesions in rats by soy flakes, soy flour, genistein, and calcium. *Am J Clin Nutr* 1998; **68**: 1394S–9S.

27. *Adlercreutz H, Epidemiology of phytoestrogens. *Baillière's Clin Endocrinol Metab* 1998; **12**: 605–23.

28. Modan B, Barell V, Lubin F et al, Low-fiber intake as an etiologic factor in cancer of the colon. *J Natl Cancer Inst* 1975; **55**: 15–18.

29. *Nestle M, Animal v. plant foods in human diets and health: Is the historical record unequivocal? *Proc Nutr Soc* 1999; **58**: 211–18.

30. Lampe JW. Health effects of vegetables and fruit: assessing mechanisms of action in human experimental studies. *Am J Clin Nutr* 1999; **70**(Suppl): 475S–90S.

31. Key TJ, Fraser GE, Thorogood M et al, Mortality in vegetarians and nonvegetarians: detailed findings from a collaborative analysis of 5 prospective studies. *Am J Clin Nutr* 1999; **70**(Suppl): 516S–24S.

32. Sesink ALA, Termont DSML, Keibeuker JH et al, Red meat and colon cancer: the cytotoxic and hyperproliferative effects of dietary heme. *Cancer Res* 1999; **59**: 5704–9.

33. de Lorgeril M, Salen P, Martin J-L et al, Mediterranean dietary pattern in a randomized trial. *Arch Intern Med* 1998; **158**: 1181–7.

34. Phillips DH, Polycyclic aromatic hydrocarbons in the diet. *Mutat Res* 1999; **443**: 139–47.

35. Thomson B, Heterocyclic amine levels in cooked meat and the implication for New Zealanders. *Eur J Cancer Prev* 1999; **8**: 201–6.

36. Sinha R, Chow WH, Kulldorff M et al, Well-done, grilled red meat increases the risk of colorectal adenomas, Cancer Res 1999; **59**: 4320–4.

37. Roberts-Thomson IC, Butler WJ, Ryan P, Meat, metabolic genotypes and risk for colorectal cancer. *Eur J Cancer Prev* 1999; **8**: 207–11.

38. *Corpet DE, Stamp D, Medline A et al, Promotion of caloric microadenoma growth in mice and rats fed cooked sugar or cooked casein and fat. *Cancer Res* 1990; **50**: 6955–8.

39. *Anderson G, Cummings S, Freedman L et al, Design of the Women's Health Initiative: clinical trial and observational study. *Controlled Clin Trials* 1998; **19**: 61–109.

40. *National Academy of Sciences, National Research Council (USA), Committee on Diet and Health, *Diet and Health: Implication for Reducing Chronic Disease Risk*. Washington, DC, National Academy Press, 1989.

5 Can non-dietary and dietary agents prevent colorectal cancer?

Paul Rozen, Bernard Levin, Graeme P Young

Introduction

For more than two decades, there has been a concerted effort made to identify and evaluate chemical compounds, termed chemopreventive agents, that could prevent, inhibit, or change the course of carcinogenesis. These studies were based on observations and beliefs that certain foods or additives (e.g. green tea or garlic) had beneficial anticarcinogenic properties. In addition, there were both astute epidemiological correlations made that pointed to the anticancer chemopreventive properties of non-steroidal anti-inflammatory drugs (NSAIDs), such as aspirin, and clinical observations connecting the use of other NSAIDs to the regression of polyps in familial adenomatous polyposis (FAP) patients.

These chemopreventive drugs include medications (e.g. aspirin) that have non-chemopreventive attributes, chemicals derived from foods and believed to have anticarcinogenic properties (e.g. lycopene from tomatoes), and chemicals especially developed for their anticarcinogenic properties (e.g. sulindac sulfone). However, it is not possible to completely address this topic without including chemicals that are natural constituents of foods (e.g. calcium, vitamins, and minerals).

The sites of action and mechanisms of chemoprevention are numerous, and vary from agent to agent.[1,2] An outline of these mechanisms is given in Table 5.1.

A systematic review of mechanisms and sites of chemopreventive action, types of agents being evaluated, and results of trials is available elsewhere.[1,2] In brief, once an agent has been identified as potentially having anticancer properties, it is evaluated for its usefulness in an animal model, which is usually given a carcinogen. It is obvious that the genetic susceptibility for cancer, the gastrointestinal tract of the test animal, and the diet given are far different from those of humans, who are themselves genetically dissimilar one to another, are eating a mixed and varied diet, and are certainly not subjected deliberately to a carcinogen. If promising results are obtained from the animal model, then short-term studies are performed in humans, looking at intermediate biomarkers of response to the chemopreventive agent. These biomarkers include, for example, suppression of epithelial proliferation and/or promotion of terminal differentiation and apoptosis (programmed cell death).[3] The next step might be a clinical trial in persons at risk for developing adenomatous polyps, for example those with an ileorectal anastomosis for FAP. Randomized placebo trials in persons with sporadic adenomatous polyps are usually the last stage, since it would take too long and too large a study to evaluate each compound for its anticolorectal cancer effect[1] (Table 5.2). In this chapter, we shall refer to some of the chemopreventive agents that have been or are being evaluated clinically and could reach clinical application.

Table 5.1 *Outline of chemoprevention mechanisms*

- Inhibition and/or deactivation of possible carcinogens
- Inhibition of proliferation
- Promotion of terminal cell differentiation and/or programmed cell death (apoptosis)
- Correction of genetic damage
- Antiangiogenesis

Table 5.2 *Steps in evaluation of possible anticarcinogenic agents*

1. A clinical impression of efficacy and/or a scientific hypothesis
2. Animal studies using a carcinogen, looking for a reduction in adenoma and/or cancer occurrence
3. Human studies evaluating:
   - Epithelial proliferation
   - Side-effects and dosage needed for therapeutic effect
   - Adenoma occurrence or recurrence

Pharmaceutical drugs

There are several such drugs that were investigated or specifically developed for their chemopreventive properties.[1] They include the following.

Non-steroidal anti-inflammatory drugs (NSAIDs)

The strongest epidemiological evidence for an effect of medications in preventing colorectal cancer is for the NSAID family in general and aspirin specifically.[4] The clinical evidence is for a 50% reduction in the incidence of large-bowel cancer. However, this evidence is indirect, as a by-product of epidemiological and follow-up studies in chronic users of asprin or other non-specific cyclooxygenase (COX) inhibitors.

It is still not clear what is the dosage of aspirin needed for preventing colorectal neoplasia, and for how many years it should be given before its benefit is obtained.[5] In addition, what are the side-effects (such as gastrointestinal bleeding) that can be expected versus the benefit in reducing the likelihood of dying from cancer? This has been noted to be a concern in the elderly, who are often taking multiple medications for a variety of disorders.[6] It should be noted that even the low dose of 10mg aspirin/day significantly reduces gastric mucosal prostaglandin levels for about 5 days after the last dosage.[7] The risk for gastroduodenal bleeding is highest with piroxicam and indomethacin, intermediate with aspirin, naproxen, and diclofenac, and lowest with ibuprofen.[2] For these reasons, chronic aspirin use has not yet gained general acceptance for cancer prevention.

Cyclooxygenase 1 (COX-1) is a naturally occurring and physiologically important enzyme involved in the synthesis of prostaglandins, and is found in the kidney, brain, and gastrointestinal mucosa, where it is cytoprotective. COX-2 is induced during the inflammatory process and during the process of cellular proliferation and progression to neoplasia. Unfortunately, in order to reduce the production of prostaglandins, aspirin and the other commonly used NSAIDs, while aiming at the COX-2 that was induced by some inflammatory process, have a non-specific effect and inhibit both COX-1 and COX-2.[4,8] This non-specific inhibition can result in the loss of cytoprotection and allow damage to occur to the gastroduodenal mucosa. Studies are being carried out with specific COX-2 inhibitors and/or promoters of apoptosis and inhibitors of invasiveness and angiogenesis, which may provide a better complication–benefit ratio than that obtained with aspirin.[9] New NSAIDs that are COX-1-sparing and COX-2-specific inhibiting medications have been developed and recently marketed.[8] These include nimesulide (Mesuled,

Helsinn Healthcare, Switzerland), which has been noted to cause the side-effect of hepatotoxicity, and nabumetone (Relifex, SmithKline Beecham, UK). The highly specific COX-2 inhibitors include celecoxib (Celebrex, Searle, USA) and rofecoxib (Vioxx, Merck, USA). So far, none of these have been approved for preventing sporadic colorectal neoplasia, but trials are in progress. Nor have all their dose-dependent side-effects been fully evaluated. Celecoxib has been approved by the US Food and Drug Administration as an adjunct therapy in FAP (see Chapter 6).

There is good clinical evidence that NSAIDs such as sulindac will inhibit the growth of adenomatous polyps in the retained rectum of FAP patients.[4,8] Sulindac and its metabolite, sulindac sulfide, also inhibit cellular proliferation and promote apoptosis. However, while reducing the number and size of adenomatous polyps in familial adenomatous patients, they inhibit both COX-1 and COX-2. Unfortunately, this is an incomplete therapeutic effect, and adenomatous tissue is still present in the mucosa, and colorectal cancer can even occur while under treatment.[10] This is not unexpected, since experimental studies using a carcinogen demonstrated that the magnitude of therapeutic response depended on how early sulindac was administered in relationship to the carcinogen administration. So, in an ongoing genetic disorder such as FAP, it is very unlikely to obtain a complete therapeutic effect.

Sulindac sulfone is the second metabolite of sulindac. It has no antiprostaglandin effect, but does promote apoptosis.[11] It, too, has an effect on the number of adenomatous polyps and their growth in the retained rectum of patients with FAP. However, clinically important dose-dependent hepatotoxicity has been reported to occur. This drug is still under investigation, and is not yet marketed.

Ursodeoxycholic acid

This is a synthesized bile acid, since it is found only in minute amounts in human bile. It has pharmaceutical properties that could make it useful as a chemopreventive agent. Its administration changes the usual constitution of hepatic bile by replacing and therefore reducing the amounts of deoxycholic acid produced and reaching the large-bowel epithelium. Deoxycholic acid and fatty acids in the colon are metabolized by bacteria to products that may be damaging to the colorectal epithelium and therefore cause cellular hyperproliferation, and they themselves also have a carcinogenic potential. Ursodeoxycholic acid prevents this and colorectal cancer from occurring in the experimental animal. However, there are no published long-term large clinical studies in humans.[1,2]

DFMO

2-Difluoromethylornithine (DFMO) is an inhibitor of the synthesis of polyamines, which are important in stimulating cell proliferation. This compound reduces the risk for colorectal and other cancers in animal experiments.[1,12] In humans, toxicity studies demonstrated a dose-dependent but reversible hearing impairment.[12] This drug is now undergoing clinical trials in humans.

Oltipraz

This drug, dithiolethionine, was developed to treat schistosomiasis. In animal experiments, it inhibits carcinogenesis.[1,13] There are no published chemoprevention studies in humans.

Postmenopausal hormones

The evidence for a protective effect of estrogen replacement therapy, with or without progesterone, comes from meta-analyses of large follow-up studies in treated women.[14] There are some prospective studies that point to a protective effect, although small and possibly transient.[15] This is consistent with the observation that large-bowel cancer is slightly less common in premenopausal women than in men, and that the rates rise in postmenopausal women.

Naturally occurring agents

Fiber

In contrast to the overall conclusion that an adequate long-term intake of fiber has a role to play in preventing large-bowel neoplasia, the beneficial effect of short-term fiber supplements is less well established (see also Chapter 4). This has been evaluated by studies looking at the effect of fiber supplements on large-bowel epithelial proliferation and/or adenoma recurrence. The effect, if beneficial, was not prominent, and is dependent on the total diet constituents eaten.[16,17]

Calcium

This mineral has been extensively investigated epidemiologically, experimentally, and clinically for its anticancer properties. Its importance as a long-term dietary factor in colorectal cancer prevention is discussed in Chapter 4. Here, we shall consider its usefulness as a pharmaceutical agent.

The strongest evidence for its use as a chemopreventive agent comes from the trial by Baron et al,[18] giving calcium or placebo to adenomatous polyp patients for 4 years. There was a small, but significantly reduced risk for adenomatous polyp recurrence in the intervened group. The daily dosage used, 3 g of calcium carbonate, added 1200 mg of calcium ion to the daily intake of dietary calcium.

Other studies used a slightly higher dose of calcium carbonate so as to provide 1500 mg of calcium ion per day. The sources of calcium used and whether they were insoluble or soluble salts did not seem to be important, and the different compounds gave similar results. Only a small proportion of ingested calcium, about 30–40%, is absorbed, and the remainder reaches the large bowel, mixed with the intestinal contents, makes some contact with the mucosa, and finally is lost in the stools. So, there is evidence that 4–6 calcium carbonate tablets/day, each providing 300 mg of calcium ion, is a dosage proven to suppress the risk for colorectal neoplasia in persons having had an adenomatous polyp, and/or large-bowel epithelial proliferation in persons having had an adenoma or family history of colorectal cancer.[1,18,19] No such studies have been performed, however, in the average-risk population.

Because of the mounting evidence supporting the beneficial effect of calcium in preventing colorectal neoplasia and other more common disorders in high-risk persons, there is greater concerted public health action to supplement diets with more calcium. The recommended intake of calcium ion for mature adults has now been increased to 1200 mg/day. However, very few people in the USA have this intake.[20] There are now a number of low-fat, high-calcium, dairy and breakfast-food products that are being marketed and gaining popularity for the prevention of osteoporosis. Calcium should be given together with suitable dietary counseling so as to provide a well-balanced diet (see also Chapter 4).[19] Contraindications to giving calcium supplements or for increasing the dietary calcium intake include hypercalcemia, nephrolithiasis, renal insufficiency, and intolerance to treatment.

Vitamins
Vitamin D

This vitamin, independently and/or with calcium, has been identified by epidemiological and experimental studies as preventing colorectal cancer.[1,2] It inhibits cellular proliferation and promotes terminal differentiation. Because of the hypercalcemia that natural vitamin D can induce, there is little clinical evidence available to prove its therapeutic usefulness. New analogues of vitamin D have been synthesized that are without its hypercalcemic effects, but maintain its antineoplastic properties. No results from large long-term clinical studies are available.[1]

β-Carotene, vitamin A and other retinoids

These inhibit cellular proliferation and induce terminal cellular differentiation in experimental models.[1] Their antioxidant properties help trap organic free radicals and deactivate excited oxygen molecules, and so prevent tissue damage. However, short-term clinical studies did not demonstrate a clear beneficial effect on adenoma recurrence or colorectal cancer incidence. This is in contrast to their beneficial effect on promoting differentiation of myeloid and squamous cells. Significant side-effects have been reported to occur with retinoids, and limit their usefulness.[2]

Folic acid

This is important for normal cellular and genetic methylation, which helps in maintaining genetic stability.[21] In humans, there is some epidemiological evidence that colorectal adenomas and cancers are more common in those persons having a low folate intake.[1,2,22] An interesting observation was made that ulcerative colitis patients, who often have a low vegetable and fruit intake, were more likely to have colorectal cancer if they were taking salazopyrine (a medication known to reduce blood levels of folic acid). A retrospective study of ulcerative colitis patients taking folic acid supplements demonstrated a reduced risk for dysplasia.[23] Even so, there are no published large-scale chemopreventive studies in humans that prove the usefulness of folic acid as an anticancer agent.

Multivitamin and mineral preparations

The antioxidant vitamins C and E have the biochemical potential and epidemiological evidence to be useful anticarcinogens, and this is also true for selenium.[1,22,24,25] The evidence from intervention studies that each, individually, has an important role to play has not been shown conclusively in humans. For this reason, they have often been given together, or with others such as β-carotene and calcium, in adenoma intervention trials. The results have not been consistently beneficial or convincing, but they are unlikely to be harmful.[1,2,26]

Bioactive drugs

These are some of the purified active principles found in fruits, vegetables, cereals, and spices, and believed to have anticancer properties (see also Chapter 4). There are many such drugs, and they were searched for, identified, and extracted from their basic natural sources. The evidence for their value was initially based on local beliefs, clinical impressions, and some epidemiological evidence. The strongest epidemiological anticancer evidence is probably for green tea or soybeans, since their intake in the Japanese population has been long-term and extensive. In Europe, the drinking of red wine has been associated epidemiologically with reduced risks for cardiovascular disease and for cancer.

These active principles have been evaluated in cancer cell cultures and experimental studies in animals. They include perillyl alcohol and limonene from citrus fruits, resveratrol from red grapes, diallyl disulfide from garlic, lycopene from tomatoes, curcumin from turmeric, flavanols from green tea, isoflavones such as genistein from soya, dithiolthiones from cruciferous vegetables, squalene from olive oil, and ferulic and phytic acids from rice bran.[27–35]

Genistein which has been widely discussed in the published literature, has a molecular structure similar to the steroid estrogen, and is therefore termed a phytoestrogen. Its modes of action are at multiple sites, and include inhibition of proliferation, promotion of apoptosis, and inhibition of angiogenesis in experimental studies, as well as an antiestrogenic effect. Its anticancer effect is in both hormone-dependent cancers (such as breast) and colon cancer. The epidemiological evidence for its preventing colorectal cancer is not as convincing as for the hormone-dependent neoplasia.[32]

Which chemopreventive agent to choose?

The drug needs to be a medication or food additive taken over the long term, having no significant side-effects, and having clinically proven cancer preventive properties (Tables 5.3 and 5.4).

From the list of medications, the new COX-2 inhibitors seem most promising. However, they still need long-term studies to be proven effective in preventing colorectal neoplasia. In addition, there has been a suggestion that their therapeutic benefit may be improved by combination therapy with drugs acting through different pathways.[36–38]

Table 5.3 Characteristics needed for a chemopreventive agent

- **Safe** – proven by long-term experimental and clinical follow-up studies
- **Effective** – proven by long-term experimental and clinical follow-up studies
- **Cheap** – for mass use
- **Easy to take** – possibly as a dietary supplement

Table 5.4 *Chemopreventive agents being evaluated and their efficacy in preventing colorectal neoplasia (see text for details)*

Agents	Mechanism of action	Evidence of efficacy		Safety
		Experimental	Clinical	
NSAIDs	Inhibit proliferation	Good	Good	Moderate
Fiber	Interaction with intraluminal contents	Good	Low	Good
Calcium	Inhibits proliferation	Good	Moderate	Good
Vitamins and minerals	Antioxidants Correct genetic damage Inhibit proliferation	Moderate	Inconsistent	Good
Bioactive drugs	Antioxidants Correct genetic damage Inhibit proliferation	Good	Epidemiological evidence; no completed trials	Good
Pharmaceuticals	Antioxidants Correct genetic damage Inhibit proliferation Promote apoptosis	Good	No completed trials	Variable

It is very likely that they will initially be made available for use in persons at increased risk for colorectal neoplasia. These include those with a strong family history of colorectal cancer or personal history of adenoma. For women, the decision to take postmenopausal replacement hormones is individual. The side-effects and long-term risks for other malignancies need to be considered.

If they are taken, then the risk for large-bowel cancer is slightly reduced.

Based on the evidence from soybean ingestion and green tea consumption, their active principles are worthy of further studies in humans at risk for colorectal cancer. In the meantime, calcium-enriched foods would seem to be useful, at a minimal risk for side-effects.

References (*Reviews and general articles)

1. *Kelloff GF, Boone CW, Sigman K et al, Chemoprevention of colorectal cancer. In: *Prevention and Early Detection of Colorectal Cancer* (Young GP, Rozen P, Levin B, eds). London: Saunders, 1996: 115–40.
2. *Langman M, Boyle F, Chemoprevention of colorectal cancer (Review). *Gut* 1998; **43:** 578–85.
3. *Boone CW, Kelloff GJ, Steele VE, Natural history of intraepithelial neoplasia in humans with implications for cancer chemoprevention strategy. *Cancer Res* 1992; **52:** 1651–9.
4. *Shiff SJ, Rigas B, Nonsteroidal anti-inflammatory drugs and colorectal cancer: evolving concepts of their chemopreventive actions. *Gastroenterology* 1997; **113:** 1992–8.
5. Collet J-P, Sharpe C, Belzile E et al, Colorectal cancer prevention by non-steroidal anti-inflammatory drugs: effects of dosage and timing. *Br J Cancer* 1999; **81:** 62–8.
6. *Koutsos MI, Shiff SJ, Rigas B, Can nonsteroidal anti-inflammatory drugs be recommended to prevent colon cancer in high-risk elderly patients? *Drugs Aging* 1995; **6:** 421–5.
7. Cryer B, Feldman M, Effects of very low dose daily, long-term aspirin therapy on gastric, duodenal and rectal prostaglandin levels and on mucosal injury in healthy humans. *Gastroenterology* 1999; **117:** 17–25.
8. Williams CS, Smalley W, Dubois RN, Aspirin use and potential mechanisms for colorectal cancer prevention. *J Clin Invest* 1997; **100:** 1325–9.
9. Dannenberg AJ, Zakim D, Chemoprevention of colorectal cancer through inhibition of cyclooxygenase-2. *Semin Oncol* 1999; **26:** 499–504.

10. Lynch HT, Thorson AG, Smyrk TC, Rectal cancer after prolonged sulindac chemoprevention. *Cancer* 1995; **75**: 936–8.

11. Piazza GA, Rahm AK, Finn TS et al, Apoptosis primarily accounts for the growth-inhibitory properties of sulindac metabolites and involves a mechanism that is independent of cyclooxygenase inhibition, cell cycle arrest and p53 induction. *Cancer Res* 1997; **57**: 2452–9.

12. *Love RR, Jacoby R, Newton MA et al, A randomized placebo-controlled trial of low-dose α-difluoromethyl-ornithine in individuals at risk for colorectal cancer. *Cancer Epidemiol Biomark Prev* 1998; **7**: 989–92.

13. Clapper ML, Chemopreventive activity of oltipraz. *Pharmacol Ther* 1998; **78**: 17-27.

14. *Grodstein F, Newcomb PA, Stampfer MJ, Postmenopausal hormone therapy and the risk of colorectal cancer: a review and meta-analysis. *Am J Med* 1999; **106**: 574–82.

15. Jacobs EJ, White E, Weiss NS et al, Hormone replacement therapy and colon cancer among members of a health maintenance organization. *Epidemiology* 1999; **10**: 445–51.

16. *Kim Y-I, AGA technical review: impact of dietary fiber on colon cancer occurrence. *Gastroenterology* 2000; **18**: 1235–57.

17. Alberts DS, Martinez ME, Roe DJ et al, Lack of effect of a high-fiber cereal supplement on the recurrence of colorectal adenomas. *N Engl J Med* 2000; **342**: 1156–62.

18. Baron JA, Beach M, Mandel JS et al, Calcium supplements for prevention of colorectal adenomas. *N Engl J Med* 1999; **340**: 101–7.

19. Rozen P, Lubin F, Papo N et al, Calcium supplements interact significantly with long-term diet while suppressing rectal epithelial proliferation of adenoma patients. *Cancer* 2001; **91**: 833–40.

20. Miller GD, Anderson JJB, The role of calcium in prevention of chronic diseases. *J Am Coll Nutr* 1999; **18**: 371S–2S.

21. *Giovannucci E, Stampfer MJ, Colditz GA et al, Multivitamin use, folate, and colon cancer in women in the Nurses' Health Study. *Ann Intern Med* 1998; **129**: 517–24.

22. Tseng M, Murray SC, Kupper LL et al, Micronutrients and the risk of colorectal adenomas. *Am J Epidemiol* 1996; **144**: 1005–14.

23. Lashner BA, Provencher KS, Seidner DL et al, The effect of folic acid supplementation on the risk for cancer or dysplasia in ulcerative colitis. *Gastroenterology* 1997; **112**: 29–32.

24. Bostick RM, Potter JD, McKenzie DR et al, Reduced risk of colon cancer with high intake of vitamin E: the Iowa Women's Health Study. *Cancer Res* 1993; **53**: 4230–7.

25. Combs, GF Jr, Gray WP, Chemopreventive agents: selenium. *Pharmacol Ther* 1998; **79**: 179–92.

26. Patterson RE, Kristal AR, Newhouser ML, Vitamin supplements and cancer risk. Epidemiologic research and recommendations. In: *Primary and Secondary Preventive Nutrition* (Bendich A, Decklebaum RJ, eds). Totowa, NJ: Humana Press, 2000: 21–43.

27. Crowell PL, Prevention and therapy of cancer by dietary monoterpenes. *J Nutr* 1999; **129**: 775S–8S.

28. Siegers C-P, Steffwen B, Röbke A et al, The effects of garlic preparations against human tumor cell proliferation. *Phytomedicine* 1999; **6**: 7–11.

29. Clinton SK. Lycopene: chemistry, biology, and implications for human health and disease. *Nutr Rev* 1998; **56**: 35–51.

30. Huang M-T, Newmark HL, Frenkel K, Inhibitory effects of curcumin on tumorigenesis in mice. *J Cell Biochem* 1997; **27**(Suppl): 25–34.

31. *Katiyar SK, Mukhtar H, Tea in chemoprevention of cancer: epidemiologic and experimental studies (Review). *Intl J Oncol* 1996; **8**: 221–8.

32. Booth C, Hargreaves DF, Hadfield JA et al, Isoflavones inhibit intestinal epithelial cell proliferation and induce apoptosis in vitro. *Br J Cancer* 1999; **80**: 1550–7.

33. Hecht SS, Chemoprevention of cancer by isothiocyanates, modifiers of carcinogen metabolism. *J Nutr* 1999; **129**: 768S–74S.

34. Rao CV, Newmark HL, Reddy BS, Chemopreventive effect of squalene on colon cancer. *Carcinogenesis* 1998; **19**: 287–90.

35. Mori H, Kawabata K, Yoshimi N et al, Chemopreventive effects of ferulic acid on oral and rice germ on large bowel carcinogenesis. *Anticancer Res* 1999; **19**: 3775–8.

36. Ip C, Ganther HE, Combination of blocking agents and suppressing agents in cancer prevention. *Carcinogenesis* 1991; **12**: 365–7.

37. Chinery R, Beauchamp RD, Shyr Y et al, Antioxidants reduce cyclooxygenase-2 expression, prostaglandin production, and proliferation in colorectal cancer cells. *Cancer Res* 1998; **58**: 2323–7.

38. Jacoby RF, Cole CE, Tutsch K et al, Chemopreventive efficacy of combined piroxicam and difluo-romethylornithine treatment of Apc mutant Min mouse adenomas, and selective toxicity against Apc mutant embryos. *Cancer Res* 2000; **60**: 1864–70.

6 Who are at risk for familial colorectal cancer and how can they be managed?

Paul Rozen, Bernard Levin, Graeme P Young

Introduction

The etiology of most cases of colorectal cancer is related to diet and lifestyle habits (see Chapters 2 and 4). However, in about 15% of cases, there is a family history of colorectal cancer and/or other malignancies (Figure 6.1). This includes a small number (<5%) where there is a recognizable dominant familial risk factor. In a larger number (>10%), there is a familial clustering of cancers and/or adenomatous polyps, which could be from a genetic susceptibility due to low-penetrance genes, or shared environmental–lifestyle risk factors, or an interaction between these two etiological causes. For an introduction to colon cancer genetics, see reference 1. References 1–3 provide an overview of the clinical features discussed below.

How to identify families at risk for colorectal cancer?

Asking a simple question 'Has anyone had cancer in your family?' can quite easily identify these families. An affirmative answer leads to the follow-up questions: 'Who has had cancer – parents, siblings, or children (first-degree relatives); grandparents, grandchildren, uncles, or aunts (second-degree relatives); cousins?'; 'Where did these tumors occur – colon, breast, ovary, etc.?' and 'At what age did these occur?'. If asking these simple questions becomes routine, then they are not time-consuming and can identify families at risk for common malignancies (Table 6.1). Answers that cause the physician to suspect a familial risk factor include cancers occurring before the age of 50–55 years and/or cancers occurring in two or more first or second-degree relatives. These 'alarm' answers demand a more detailed cancer pedigree (see reference 1).

It is often useful to identify a family 'mentor(s)' who either knows the family's history or is willing and acceptable to the family to list the relatives and make initial

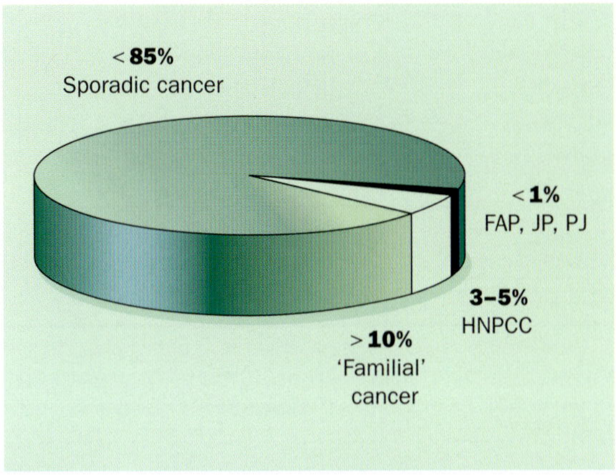

Figure 6.1 *Relative and approximate contributions of familial causes to the incidence of colorectal cancer: FAP, familial adenomatous polyposis; JP, familial juvenile polyposis; PJ, Peutz–Jeghers syndrome; HNPCC, hereditary non-polyposis colorectal cancer.*

Table 6.1 *Questions to ask for ascertaining familial cancer risk*

Has anyone had cancer in your family?
If affirmative ....

- Who had cancer?
- Where was their cancer?
- At what age did it occur?

contact with them so as to obtain permission for further questions and to obtain some medical information. This is then followed up by a sympathetic medical interviewer, who, by telephone, can ask directed questions and obtain written permission to obtain medical records, pathology reports, discharge summaries, or death certificates. A more detailed family pedigree can then be drawn up by a trained medical interviewer or experienced family physician or consultant, and/or referred to a genetic counselor or medical geneticist. This pedigree allows the visualization of the pathways of inheritance and patterns of disease (organ-specific or distribution of neoplasia among organs) that may be consistent with a specific genetic disorder.

How to classify families at risk for colorectal cancer?

These families fall into three categories, in descending order of risk for cancer. The first group has the smallest number of cases, and includes those having recognizable genetic syndromes: The second is a larger group having a strong familial history of colorectal cancer and/or other neoplasia, but not initially identifiable as belonging to a defined syndrome. The third and largest number includes the first-degree relatives of persons who have had sporadic colorectal cancer (Table 6.2).

The defined genetic syndromes

Many years of astute clinical observations and recent progress in cancer genetics have defined easily recognizable but uncommon cancer syndromes, as those with or without antecedent large-bowel polyps of adenomatous or other histological types. The number of polyps and their histology, and the clinical manifestations of the disease, which almost always include extracolonic involvement, help classify the syndromes.

Table 6.2 *Classifying causes of familial risk for colorectal cancer and their relative contributions to the total cancer burden*

Defined genetic syndromes

- With many adenomatous polyps
  - Familial adenomatous polyposis (<1%)
- With hamartomatous polyps
  - Familial juvenile polyposis (<1%)
  - Peutz–Jeghers syndrome (<1%)
- With few adenomatous polyps
  - Hereditary non-polyposis colorectal cancer (3–5%)
  - Ethnic-specific susceptibility polymorphisms (?)

Undefined familial risk

- First-degree relatives of colon cancer or adenoma patients (>10%)

Familial syndromes characterized by intestinal polyposis

These syndromes are classified clinically as having multiple adenomatous polyps or non-neoplastic, hamartomatous polyps (Figure 6.2).

Familial adenomatous polyposis (FAP)

This condition is described in detail here, since it illustrates the overall clinical problem of familial cancer.[4]

The classical clinical definition of FAP is based on the finding of more than 100 colonic adenomatous polyps. This is an autosomal (not sex-related) dominant condition that occurs in one of 5–10 000 births. The polyps usually appear at the time of adolescence and thereafter increase in numbers; if the patient is an affected carrier, the polyps are usually found by the age of 40 years. Colonic cancer occurs inevitably and at an earlier than usual age, but only rarely before the age of 20 years.[4,5] There are gastrointestinal extracolonic manifestations of disease, which include gastric polyps (mostly non-adenomatous 'fundic gland' polyps) and small-bowel adenomas, both of which rarely require intervention. However, duodenal adenomas, especially those on or around the papilla of Vater, may grow to a large size, undergo progressive dysplasia, and become invasive carcinomas (Figure 6.3).[4] Extra-intestinal manifestations include subcutaneous tumors, osteomas, and dental abnormalities – none of which are malignant – and soft-tissue ('desmoid') tumors in the mesentery or areas of scars that are benign, but locally can form life-threatening masses. Gardner described the presence of these extra-intestinal lesions, and this phenotypic variant is named after him.[2] Retinal pigmented spots (congenital hypertrophy of the retinal epithelium) are found in a number of cases, but are not diagnostic of FAP. Other rare lesions include thyroid or liver or brain tumors.

The genetic etiology of FAP has been identified as a mutation occurring on chromosome 5q in the area of the *APC* gene.[3] Many mutations have been identified, and, in general, there is a correlation between the genetic site and the severity of clinical manifestation.[3,5–7] Laboratory success in identifying the mutation is about 70–90%, but requires the DNA of an affected patient.[8] This identification is important, since it can be used as a screening test for possible mutation carriers in the asymptomatic family members at risk.[8,9]

Diagnosis

This is essentially dependent on the clinical suspicion of the physician, and, whenever possible, it should be confirmed by genetic analysis. Genetic testing of children at

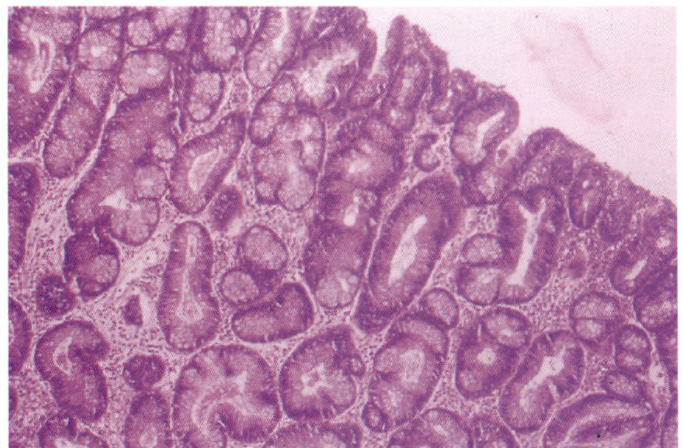

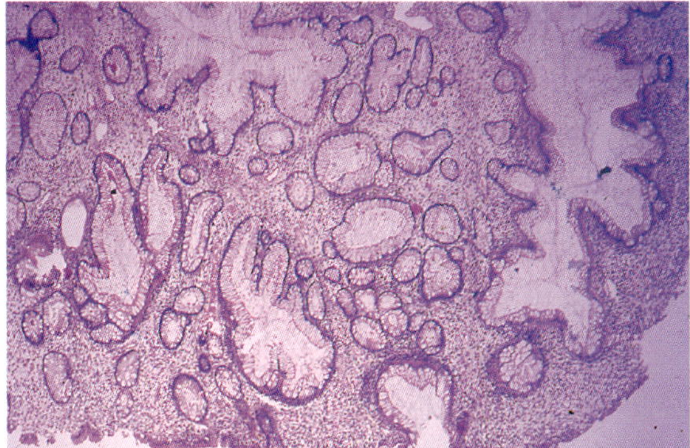

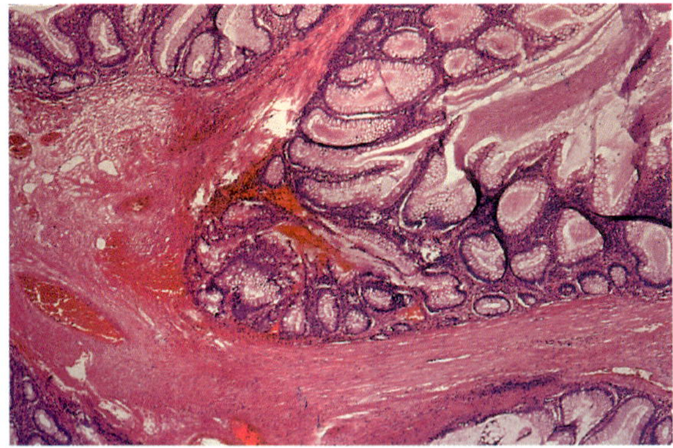

Figure 6.2 *(a) Section from a typical adenomatous polyp. Note the tubular morphology of the crypts, and the dark-stained elongated nuclei indicative of mild dysplasia. (b) Section from a juvenile polyp. These are red, round, smooth, or lobulated polyps. Microscopically, they are characterized by cystic dilatation of mucus-containing glands lined by normal epithelium. There is often a dense inflammatory infiltration of the stoma and no bands of smooth muscle in the lamina propria. (c) Section from a Peutz–Jeghers polyp. The histological appearance of this hamartomatous polyp is similar to that of the juvenile polyp, other than the typical presence of bands of smooth muscle in the lamina propria.*

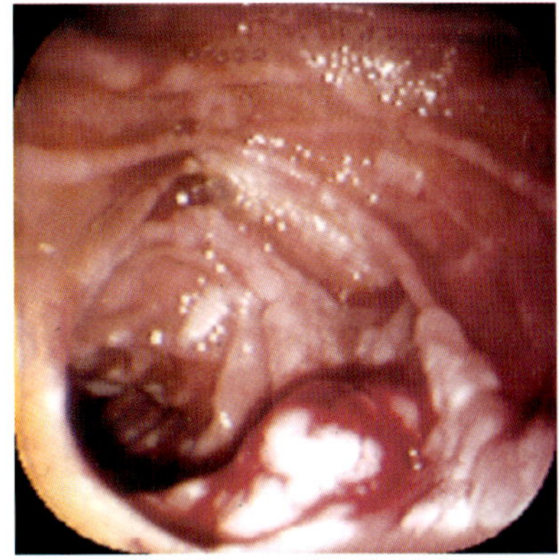

Figure 6.3 *Large bleeding duodenal adenoma in a FAP patient. Small flat adenomas are seen in the adjacent mucosa.*

risk is performed just before or at puberty, when the diagnosis becomes of clinical relevance. The mutation-negative child can then be left without further investigation. The mutation-positive child (or all children, if no mutation can be identified in the FAP patient, or if no patient is available for testing) is best seen by the examining gastroenterologist, and the child or youth is given an explanation about the necessity for an intrarectal examination. At the first examination, it is best to do a brief and minimal flexible sigmoidoscopy with directed and random biopsies. A painful or psychologically traumatic endoscopy reduces the chances of gaining cooperation for a more complete examination in the future. The child or young adult should be seen and followed up by the one physician with whom the patient feels comfortable. The child is easily frightened and anxious, especially when the family history of cancer and operations are discussed. Once the youth's confidence is obtained, then, at about the age of completing secondary schooling, a baseline colonoscopic examination should be performed. This might be needed earlier if there are symptoms or multiple polyps found at sigmoidoscopy or there was a family history of colorectal cancer at an early age.[5]

Recently, it has become apparent that the clinical features may not be 'classical', and there may be relatively few or even no large-bowel adenomas at the time of endoscopic examination, or they may occur only in the proximal colon. This condition has been called 'attenuated' FAP. In this context, when FAP is suspected, colonoscopy is therefore the best way to pursue the diagnosis. The adenomas may be small and flat or may be intramucosal, and are therefore identified by taking multiple random biopsies or by dye-staining and using a magnifying colonoscope. Histologically, these are called 'microadenomas' (Figure 6.4).[2,6,10]

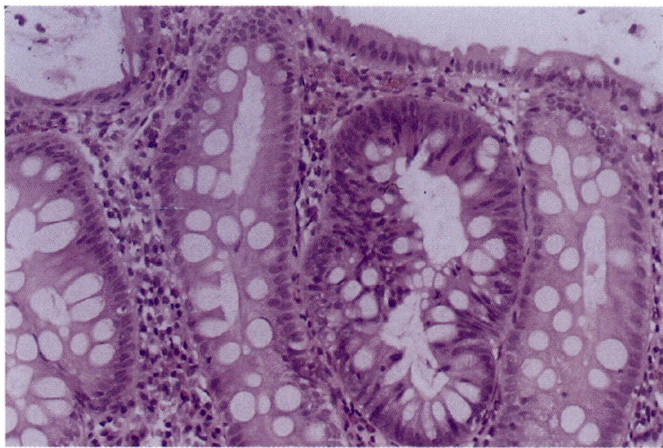

Figure 6.4 *Microadenoma. Note the appearance of dark-stained and elongated nuclei in a distorted crypt that does not protrude above the surrounding normal surface epithelium.*

The treating physician needs to be aware that the clinical manifestations of FAP may vary between family members and between branches of that extended, but affected family (Table 6.3).[7] Thus, a one-time clinical examination does not necessarily exclude FAP. If genetic testing is unavailable, then the at-risk family members must continue to be under close systematic clinical and endoscopic follow-up.

As stated, large-bowel endoscopy is the most important clinical examination. However, the disease is lifelong and there are multiple clinical manifestations.[1,4] An annual physical examination includes an evaluation for soft-tissue or bone lesions or abdominal masses. Abdominal ultrasound examination, gastroduodenoscopy, and colonoscopy are performed before elective surgery of the colon (Table 6.4).

Treatment

This is by surgical removal of the large intestine, before cancer occurs. The usual age for this is the late teens or early twenties.[4] As this is usually an elective procedure, the timing can be arranged so as to be least inconvenient,

Table 6.3 *Phenotypic variations in familial adenomatous polyposis*

- Between families having the same site of mutation (interfamilial variation)
- Between members of same family (intrafamilial variation)

The assumption is that there are unrecognized modifying genes and/or genetic–environmental interactions

for example during vacation before starting studies or a new job. For young women, it is sometimes best arranged either before marriage or after pregnancies. The elective surgery can be further delayed if there is good rapport with a compliant patient and the polyps are sparse and not large.[4,7,11] The most common reasons for delaying surgery are a desire to complete a study program or the family. This requires careful clinical and colonoscopic annual follow-up. The surgical treatment is usually removal of the entire large bowel, stripping the remaining rectal mucosa down to the dentate line and forming an internal pouch from the small intestine.[4,12,13] This is usually a two-stage procedure with a temporary diverting ileostomy. However, there are medical centers that perform this at one stage, which is obviously more convenient for the patient but problematic if there is an anastomatic leak. In a few cases, where there are sparse polyps, a low ileorectal anastomosis is performed, leaving rectal mucosa for careful biannual endoscopic follow-up.[13]

Follow-up

It is essential that annual follow-up continues after the surgical procedures have been completed.[14] This includes physical examination, abdominal ultrasound, and computed tomography (CT) or magnetic resonance imaging (MRI) if there is a suspected desmoid tumor. Upper endoscopy with a gastroscope, alternating with a side-viewing duodenscope, should be performed every 1–3 years in order to identify peri- and ampullary duodenal adenomas.[14,15] These polyps should be ablated endoscopically before they reach a large size and/or become invasive cancers (Figure 6.3 and Table 6.4).

Chemoprevention

There are no agreed upon chemopreventive recommendations for FAP patients with an intact colon.[16] However, non-steroidal anti-inflammatory drugs (NSAIDs), including the selective cyclooxygenase-2 (COX-2) inhibitors, suppress adenoma growth, and they provide supplemental treatment to endoscopic polypectomy if there is an intact rectum post colectomy. The treatment can be in the form of suppositories or medications by mouth. However, there are case reports of rectal cancer occurring even without polyp growth. So, in some cases, this is only a temporizing treatment before definitive surgery (see Chapter 5). Based on the results of a multicenter placebo-controlled trial, there is now US Federal Drug Administration (FDA) approval to use the selective COX-2 inhibitor celecoxib as a supplemental treatment, for reducing the adenomatous polyp burden, even in the intact colon of FAP patients (Figure 6.5). Its longer-term usefulness remains to be evaluated.[17]

Table 6.4 *Screening for familial adenomatous polyposis*

Diagnosis
DNA testing, pre- or postnatal, is useful in over 70% of cases. If it is positive or not available, then the following should be done:
- Flexible sigmoidoscopy at age 10–12 years with random mucosal biopsies
- Colonoscopy with random biopsies at age 18–20 years; repeated every 2 years
- Retinal examinations to identify congenital hypertrophy of the retinal pigment epithelium (CHRPE) (elective test)
- Panoramic X-rays of face for osteomas (elective test)

Follow-up
- Yearly physical examination
- Yearly ultrasound of abdomen (elective test)
- Rectal surveillance, every 3–12 months, if ileorectal anastomosis was performed
- Gastroscopy or duodenoscopy, alternating every 1–3 years

There is no established chemopreventive or therapeutic protocol for desmoid tumors. In some cases, desmoid tumors regress or do not progress in size. These are best left alone, since any surgical procedure can stimulate further growth or recurrence. Desmoids occurring in the abdominal wall may require surgical removal if bulky. An antiestrogen (tamoxifen) and NSAIDs have been tried when there is evidence of desmoid tumor progression, and have been found useful. There are also case reports of success with other medications.[18]

Prognosis and support
After colectomy, FAP patients may die from rectal cancer, if an ileorectal anastomosis was performed, or desmoid tumors or duodenal cancers, or from other rare complications.[14] They need lifelong medical and emotional support. There are often intrafamilial crises if the marriage partner has not been prepared adequately by a genetic counselor. Affected children who have not been adequately counseled may develop antagonistic feelings towards the disease-transmitting parent. They may need help from an understanding child psychologist.[2]

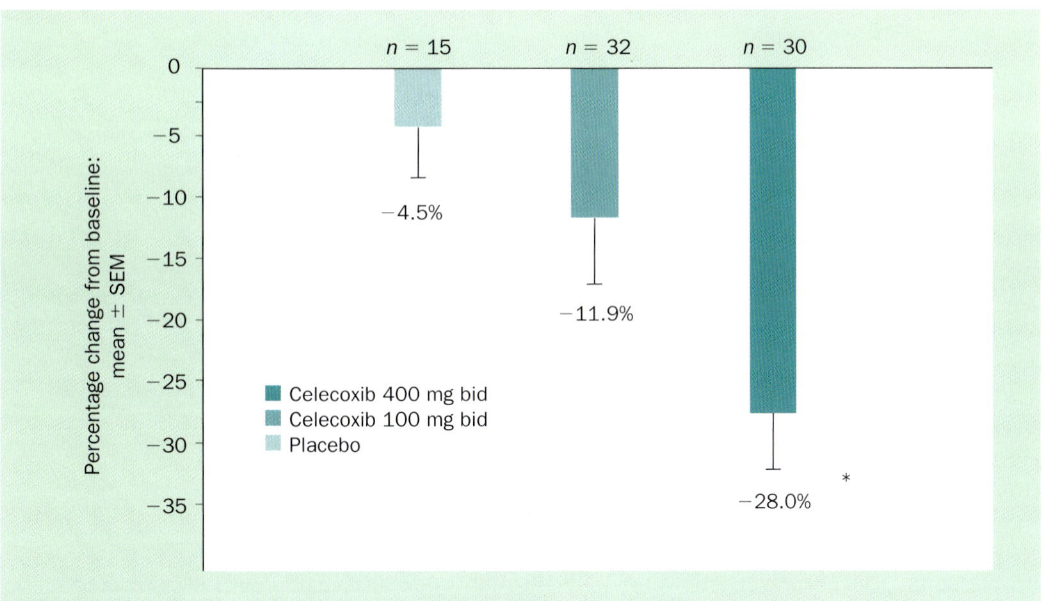

Figure 6.5 *Change in the number of colorectal polyps in FAP patients receiving placebo or celecoxib (Celebrex) for 6 months. The reduction in polyp burden was highly significant (*p = 0.003 versus placebo) with the dosage of 400 mg twice a day. Figure derived from reference 17 and published with permission of the authors.*

The hamartomatous polyposis syndromes

These include familial juvenile polyposis and Peutz–Jeghers syndrome. They must be differentiated from FAP, since their clinical manifestations, genetic diagnosis, treatment, follow-up, and prognosis are different.[1–3] The essential diagnostic element is the polyp histology (Figure 6.2). An experienced gastrointestinal histopathologist is needed for making this differential diagnosis. Even so, there may still be some confusion in classification, since the histology may show a 'mixed' picture, which includes adenomatous or other elements. These may be part of the syndrome ('mixed adenomatous–juvenile polyps') or dysplastic changes occurring in the progression of the hamartoma to malignancy.[19,20]

Familial juvenile polyposis

Sporadic colonic juvenile polyps are a common finding in infants, sometimes causing symptoms, but usually occurring without a family history of polyps or cancer. The familial syndrome is uncommon, and there the polyps can be found not only in the colon but also in the stomach and small intestine. The clinical features may also include non-gastrointestinal lesions, and these have led to a subclassification into other syndromes: Cowden, Bannayan–Ruvalcaba–Riley, and Gorlin.[21] This, and the different mutations that have been identified, led to the realization that familial juvenile polyposis is a heterogeneous condition – that is, different mutations can cause the appearance of juvenile polyps and the various other clinical manifestations.[21,22]

It has been estimated that in familial juvenile polyposis, there is a 50% lifetime risk for cancer and a 15% risk for colon cancer.[21] Patients and their affected first-degree relatives need repeated routine physical examination and upper and lower endoscopy. Small-bowel radiological examination and enteroscopy need to be performed if there is a suspicion of small-bowel polyps. Whenever possible, endoscopic polypectomy should be performed, and surgery delayed until the clinical features, the number of polyps, and their dysplastic changes require surgical intervention. The surgical procedure should be tailored to answer the clinical need, since, in contrast to FAP, where definitive surgery is recommended because of the high risk for colorectal cancer and where each surgical procedure can lead to adhesions and desmoid tumors, this is not the case in familial juvenile polyposis.[23] Intraoperative enteroscopy will then be useful to identify and treat small-bowel lesions.[24]

Mutations causing syndromes having juvenile polyps have been identified on chromosomes 6, 9, 10, and 18. Identifying the particular mutation is difficult, but, if successful, it becomes a useful screening test for that particular family.[22]

Peutz–Jeghers syndrome

This is an uncommon genetic disorder, having about one-third of the incidence of FAP. However, it is easily identified clinically by the pigmented spots that appear on the lips and other mucous membranes such as the buccal mucosa, nail beds, conjunctiva, palms, and soles.[1,25] The pigmentation can be identified during infancy, but may fade away by early adulthood. The polyps have a characteristic histology and are not neoplastic; however, dysplasia can occur and leads to cancer (Figure 6.2). The polyps can occur throughout the gastrointestinal tract, and even in other organs. The clinical complaints are often related to obstruction or bleeding of the gastrointestinal tract. The risk for cancer in the gastrointestinal tract and elsewhere is high by early–mid adulthood. Cancers occur in the gastrointestinal tract, pancreas, breasts, uterus, ovaries, and testes.[26]

Because of the pleomorphic manifestations and sites of neoplasia, repeated medical examinations are needed, starting from early adulthood. These include physical examination, breast, gynecological, and testicular examinations, and abdominal ultrasonography. Other tests include gastrointestinal endoscopy to identify and remove polypoid lesions, and small-intestinal radiological examination and enteroscopy to examine the small intestine especially when surgery is performed. Genetically, this syndrome has a high degree of penetrance, and in many cases, the mutation has been found on chromosome 19.[25,27]

Other non-adenomatous polyposis syndromes

These include hyperplastic polyposis with a risk for familial colorectal cancer and the Cronkhite–Canada syndrome. The latter syndrome is not familial, but is also associated with a risk for colorectal cancer.[1] The hyperplastic polyps themselves are not precancerous, but the overall condition is.

Familial syndromes not characterized by many intestinal polyps

Adenomatous polyps can occur in these conditions, but they are usually few in number.[1]

Hereditary non-polyposis colorectal cancer (HNPCC)

This is probably the most commonly occurring defined genetic syndrome, contributing to about 5% of all colorectal cancers. Warthin recognized it as a cause of familial cancer, but Henry Lynch defined its clinical features and recognized its clinical importance as an example of familial cancer that could be helped by early recognition and surgical treatment[1,3,28] – hence the synonym 'Lynch syndrome'.

It is a dominant disorder with a high degree of penetrance, although 'skipped generations' can occur. The genetic pathway to neoplasia is uniquely different from that of sporadic large-bowel cancer. The commonest mutations occur on chromosomes 2 (*MSH2*) and 3 (*MLH1*), and there are at least four others; they allow 'naturally occurring' errors in chromosome replication to remain uncorrected, and this is termed defective mismatch repair. This pathway allows cancer to appear relatively quickly in young adulthood.[28–30]

The cancer commonly occurs in the colon without the appearance of precusor adenomatous polyps – hence its name. However, adenomatous polyps may be found, but not in large numbers. There is a high likelihood of the cancer appearing in other gastrointestinal and non-gastrointestinal organs, with or without colonic involvement.[29] These include the small intestine, pancreas, ovary, uterus, urinary tract, skin, and brain, and there is a higher risk for breast cancer and stomach cancer in some families.

In this syndrome, the appearance of a brain tumor is called the Turcot syndrome. The concurrent occurrence of sebaceous tumors of the skin and a small-bowel and/or other tumors is called the Muir–Torre syndrome (Figure 6.6).[1,28,30]

Diagnosis

As there is no diagnostic phenotype or easily performed screening test, the initial diagnosis is clinical.[31] This has been defined as follows:

- there must be two generations with cancer involving three or more relatives from the same family, one of whom should be younger than 50 years of age;
- one of the cancers should be of the colon and the others might be of the other HNPCC target organs.[30]

These are referred to as the 'modified Amsterdam criteria'. There are affected families that do not completely fulfill these clinical criteria.[28] FAP needs to be excluded, and sometimes it is difficult to differentiate HNPCC from attenuated FAP.

The identification of the actual mutation is difficult because of the large number of genetic sites at risk. If found, it is obviously very useful as a screening test of the relatives at risk. However, there are other indirect tests that can help in classifying the cancer case as probably belonging to this HNPCC syndrome and can identify the genetic site of the responsible mutation. Microsatellites are repetitive sequences of DNA that are found in the chromosome, between coding areas of the gene. The genetic disturbance in HNPCC allows a disorder of these

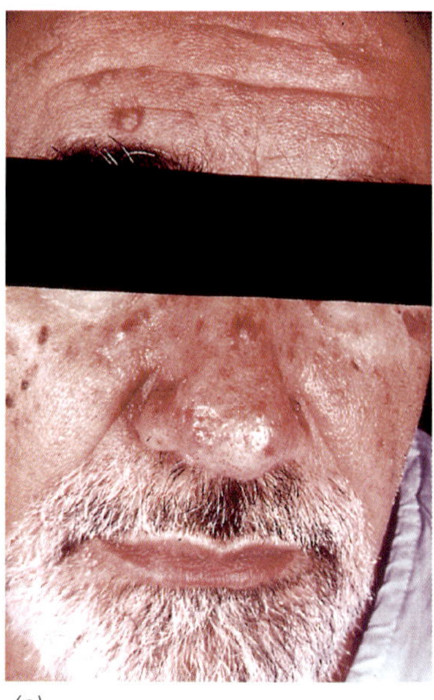

(a)

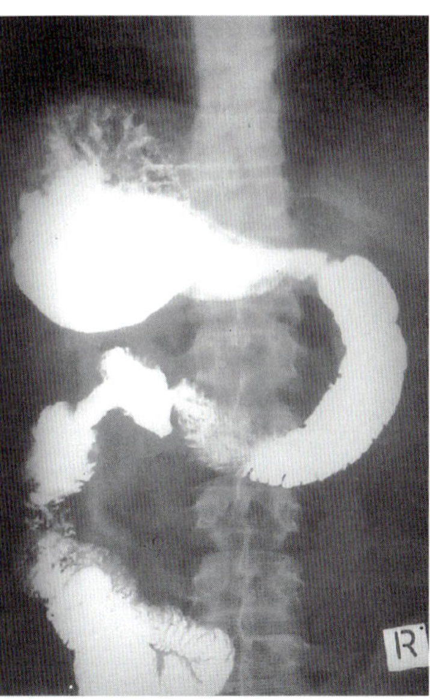

(b)

Figure 6.6 (a) *Muir–Torre syndrome: multiple sebaceous adenomas found on the face of a patient having a typical HNPCC family history.*
(b) *Upper gastrointestinal X-ray of the same patient, demonstrating a postduodenal narrowing due to a cancer of the small intestine.*

sequences to remain uncorrected, and this can be detected and quantified. The finding of a significant degree of microsatellite instability (MSI) in the tumor tissue itself ('MSI-high') is consistent with the pathogenetic pathway of HNPCC. This test is now becoming more readily available. The criteria to define MSI-high, or -low, or -stable, were established at a US National Institutes of Health (NIH) workshop held in Bethesda, Maryland. These are referred to as the 'Bethesda criteria', and they also include a broader set of clinical criteria for examining the presence of MSI.[28,29] In addition, there are now immunohistochemical tests to stain the tumor tissue and indicate whether chromosome 2 or 3 is intact or mutated. If either is not intact, then this would be consistent with a mutation in that chromosome; it could be somatic and in the tumor only – or it could be a germline mutation, in which case there is the possibility of HNPCC[32] (Figure 6.7). This is a useful, simple, and inexpensive screening test.

Screening or follow-up post operation

Screening should start about 5–10 years younger than the youngest cancer-affected relative, but no later than 40 years in the absence of genetic testing.[28] However, as neoplasia can appear in early adult life and genetic testing may not be available or informative, it is usually recommended to start screening in the early twenties.[33,34] There is also an advantage in getting the at-risk young relatives used to periodic examinations before they get diverted into other activities and responsibilities. The annual protocol should include a complete system review and physical examination; tests include a urine examination, abdominal ultrasound examination, and gynecological and breast examinations and a colonoscopic examination at least every 2 years (even after subtotal colectomy).[35] If the family history is indicative of neoplasia in other target organs (e.g. stomach), then these should also be included in the screening protocol.[28,33] This protocol of targeted screening has been shown to be cost-effective in reducing mortality from large-bowel cancer (Table 6.5).[30,34,36]

Treatment

There is no evidence at present that preventive dietary treatment changes the risk for neoplasia in these patients. However, it would seem pragmatic to advise a healthy lifestyle and dietary habits. There are no positive results available from chemopreventive trials in HNPCC patients. Only some HNPCC tumors express COX-2, and so it remains to be seen whether they would be responsive to NSAID chemoprevention.[28,37] There is also some clinical

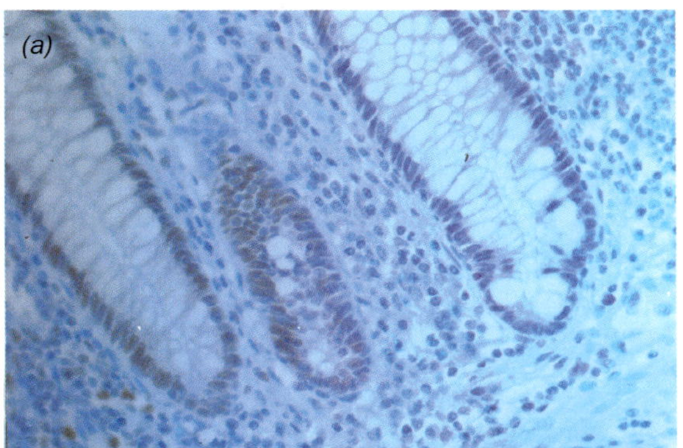

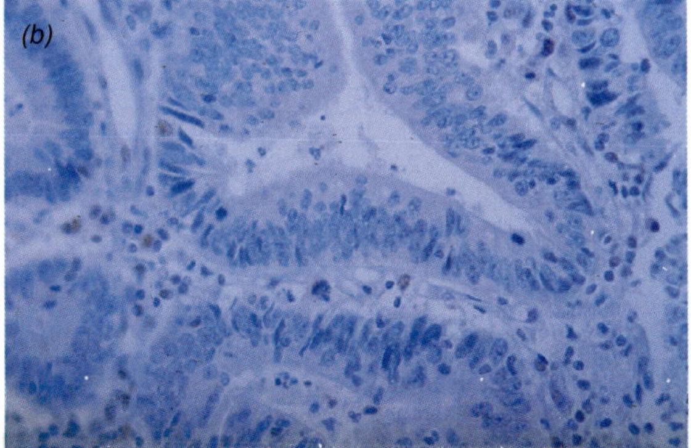

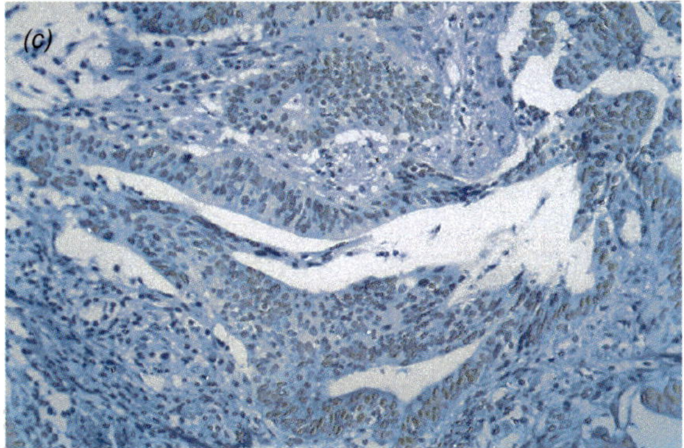

Figure 6.7 *Immunohistology of an HNPCC large-bowel cancer and adjacent normal tissue with an antibody against the MSH2 protein. (a) The non-neoplastic tissue, having an intact allele, shows normal brown nuclear staining. (b) The tumor tissue, not having an intact MSH2, does not stain at all. A few lymphocytes show normal nuclear staining. (c) The same stain, in a case of sporadic colorectal cancer, shows normal brown nuclear staining, indicating intact MSH2. (Figure provided by Dr E Brazowski, Tel Aviv.)*

and experimental evidence that HNPCC tumors are relatively resistant to 5-fluorouracil (5-FU).[38]

If neoplasia occurs, then the treatment is surgical. In the case of colonic neoplasia, the recommendation is for an extended resection so as to remove much of the target organ at risk, but also to maintain the quality of life. As neoplasia can recur, the final result might be ileorectal or ileoanal anastomosis and pouch.[35] If a female patient is menopausal and/or there is a family history of uterine–ovarian cancer, then a preventive ophorectomy and hysterectomy are recommended at the time of colonic surgery.[28]

Prognosis

It has been demonstrated that identification of mutation carriers, or even those just having the clinical criteria for HNPCC, and their prospective clinical screening will reduce their mortality from large-bowel cancer.[36] Even those persons who have had a colorectal cancer treated have a longer survival than those having the same stage of sporadic cancer.[39]

Other defined genetic susceptibility conditions

A widely prevalent but low-penetrance polymorphism (I1307K) in the *APC* gene on chromosome 5, leading to susceptibility to colorectal neoplasia, has been identified in Ashkenazi Jews, who are an ethnic group at risk for cancer.[3] This leads to an unstable *APC* gene and allows cancer to occur at a slightly higher than expected rate.[40] Its clinical use as a marker of risk has not been established. Similar low-penetrance but highly prevalent susceptibility mutations will probably be found in other ethnic groups or extended families at risk for colorectal cancer.

Relatives of colorectal neoplasia patients

Both retrospective analyses and prospective screening studies have demonstrated that first-degree relatives of 'sporadic' colorectal cancer or adenoma patients are at risk for the same neoplasia.[41–43] The degree of risk depends on the age of diagnosis of the patient's neoplasm, the number of relatives affected with colorectal neoplasia, and the age of the investigated relative.[44] As most sporadic colorectal neoplasia cannot be attributed to a defined genetic syndrome, the number of relatives at risk is very large (Figure 6.1). The range of risk, by strength of family history, can be seen in Tables 6.6 and 6.7.[44] The adult descendents at risk often have a higher degree of compliance for screening than do the patients' siblings, and they should all be encouraged to do so.

The recommended screening protocol is dependent on the estimated degree of risk for colorectal cancer, and is shown in Table 6.8.

Table 6.5 *Screening and follow-up of Lynch syndrome (HNPCC)*

Start screening from age 20 years, or 5–10 years less than the youngest first-degree cancer relative

- Yearly physical examination
- Yearly fecal occult blood test (alternating with colonoscopy) (elective test)
- Colonoscopy every 2 years, and also if after partial colonic resection
- Yearly ultrasound – abdominal and gynecological (elective test)
- Yearly urine tests (elective test)
- Breast screening
- DNA tests (useful in about 40%)

Genetic–environmental interactions and chemoprevention

As already discussed in the sections on FAP and HNPCC, the clinical manifestations of disease can vary from family to family, and even within families. This may be due to the presence of modifying genes and/or interactions with the environment, especially diet and lifestyle.[45] Chemoprevention will modify the polypoid expression of adenomas in FAP, but as yet there are no definitive published results of chemopreventive trials in FAP patients with an intact colon, or in HNPCC patients.

Diet and lifestyle are closely related to the etiology and prevention of colorectal neoplasia. At present, it would seem prudent to recommend a 'healthy' diet and lifestyle to patients at risk for colorectal neoplasia.[3,16,19,46] There is some epidemiological evidence that aspirin has an effect in reducing the risk for sporadic large-bowel cancer. Based on this, large-scale studies are being performed in adenoma patients using COX-2 inhibitors. However, as yet, there is no consensus to promote the routine use of aspirin or any other NSAID to prevent this neoplasm (see Chapters 4 and 5).

Socio-legal aspects of familial cancer and counseling

The identification of an affected high-risk patient with or without an identified genetic mutation can lead to guilt, anxiety, cancer phobia, denial, and refusal to collaborate. These patients and their families need a sympathetic treating physician who understands the complexity of their condition and can provide clear advice.[3,28,47–49] However, a

Table 6.6 Lifetime risk ratios for proband with a family history of colorectal cancer[a]

Neoplasia patient	Relative risk for colon cancer to first-degree relative
One parent with cancer	3–4
One sibling with cancer	3–7
First-degree relative with adenomatous polyp	3–4
First-degree relative age <60 years with adenoma	3.6
First-degree relative age >70 years with adenoma	1.4
Family history of colon cancer, proband with adenoma	3

[a] Derived from reference 44.

Table 6.7 Cumulative risk (%) of cancer for probands who have a first-degree relative with colon cancer as compared to the risk in a control population[a]

Age of proband (years)	Age of colon cancer relative		Control
	<55 years	>55 years	
	Risk for colon cancer (%)		
29	—	—	—
39	0.2	0.1	0.0
49	0.9	0.5	0.1
59	2.8	1.0	0.6
69	5.0	2.2	1.3
79	8.4	4.4	2.4

[a] Derived from reference 44.

Table 6.8 Screening protocol for first-degree relatives of sporadic colorectal cancer or adenoma patients

Start screening from age 40 years, or 5 years less than the youngest cancer relative
One relative aged ≥55 years with neoplasia:
- Yearly fecal occult blood test
- Flexible sigmoidoscopy every 5 years

One relative aged < 55 years with neoplasia, or more than one relative of any age:
- Yearly fecal occult blood test, between colonoscopies (elective test)
- Colonoscopy every 5 years

geneticist or genetic counselor is needed prior to genetic testing, and they are especially important when dealing with prenuptial young adults.[2] Not involving the future spouse can lead to extreme strains on intrafamilial relationships when the medical condition and risk for cancer become known. Children may need help from a psychologist who understands the medical problem, especially if they need to undergo a potentially traumatic or mutilating procedure such as creation of a stoma. As many patients may be underage, informed consent from parents must be obtained for all genetic testing and other invasive procedures.[50] It is usually recommended and required that a geneticist and not the treating physician obtain this informed consent.

Medical records need to be available and information transferable when needed. However, medical secrecy must also be maintained. The information is not only relevant to the affected patient, but also to his or her immediate family and even to future descendents. This leads to ethical dilemmas, and patients may even refuse to provide a family history or undergo diagnostic procedures.[48,49,51] A more common and difficult problem occurs when the affected patient refuses to allow the information to be provided to the unsuspecting immediate family at risk.[52] Another common problem is that identification of an asymptomatic person at risk and needing diagnosis and follow-up could lead to loss of job and of medical and life insurances.[3,28,48,49,51–54] These fears inhibit patients' cooperation. There is no simple answer to these problems, and they will probably need to be addressed by legislation.[55]

Physician compliance

This issue is rarely addressed. Medical students, family physicians, internists, surgeons, gastroenterologists, gynecologists, and oncologists must be educated about the importance of obtaining a simple family cancer history. This can lead to the identification of a family at risk for colorectal cancer who may require investigation and careful follow-up. Courts of law have now recognized that failure to obtain a relevant family history can be considered medical negligence.[48,56]

References (*Reviews and general articles)

1. *Menko FH, *Genetics of Colorectal Cancer for Clinical Practice.* Dordrecht: Kluwer, 1993.

2. *Burt RW, Peterson GM, Familial colorectal cancer. In: *Prevention and Early Detection of Colorectal Cancer* (Young GP, Rozen P, Levin B, eds). London: Saunders, 1996: 171–94.

3. *Lynch HT, Smyrk TC, Hereditary colorectal cancer. *Semin Oncol* 1999; **26**: 478–84.

4. *Bülow S, Familial adenomatous polyposis. *Ann Med* 1989; **21**: 299–307.

5. Eccles DM, Lunt PW, Wallis Y et al, An unusually severe phenotype for familial adenomatous polyposis. *Arch Dis Child* 1997; **77**: 431–5.

6. *Friedl W, Meuschel S, Caspari R et al, Attenuated familial adenomatous polyposis due to a mutation in the 3′ part of the APC gene. A clue for understanding the function of the APC protein. *Hum Genet* 1996; **97**: 579–84.

7. Rozen P, Samuel Z, Shomrat R et al, Notable intrafamilial phenotypic variability in a kindred with familial adenomatous polyposis and an *APC* mutation in exon 9. *Gut* 1999; **45**: 829–33.

8. *Gebert JF, Dupon C, Kadmon M et al, Combined molecular and clinical approaches for the identification of families with familial adenomatous polyposis coli. *Ann Surg* 1999; **229**: 350–61.

9. Bapat B, Noorani H, Cohen Z et al, Cost comparison of predictive genetic testing versus conventional clinical screening for familial adenomatous polyposis. *Gut* 1999; **44**: 698–703.

10. Kubota O, Kino I, Depressed adenomas of the colon in familial adenomatous polyposis. Histology, immunohistochemical detection of proliferating cell nuclear antigen (PCNA), and analysis of the background mucosa. *Am J Surg Pathol* 1995; **19**: 318–27.

11. *Phillips RKS, Spigelman AD, Can we safely delay or avoid prophylactic colectomy in familial adenomatous polyposis? *Br J Surg* 1996; **83**: 769–70.

12. Ziv Y, Church JM, Oakley JR et al, Results after restorative proctocolectomy and ileal pouch – anal anastomosis in patients with familial adenomatous polyposis and coexisting colorectal cancer. *Br J Surg* 1996; **83**: 1578–80.

13. *Setti-Carraro P, Nicholls RJ, Choice of prophylactic surgery for the large bowel component of familial adenomatous polyposis (Review). *Br J Surg* 1996; **83**: 885–92.

14. *Galle TS, Juel K, Bülow S, Causes of death in familial adenomatous polyposis. *Scand J Gastroenterol* 1999; **34**: 808–12.

15. Burke CA, Beck GJ, Church JM et al, The natural history of untreated duodenal and ampullary adenomas in patients with familial adenomatous polyposis followed in an endoscopic surveillance program. *Gastrointest Endosc* 1999; **49**: 358–64.

16. *Hawk E, Lubet R, Limburg P, Chemoprevention in hereditary colorectal cancer syndromes. *Cancer* 1999; **86**(Suppl): 2551–63.

17. Steinbach G, Lynch PM, Phillips RKS et al, A randomized, double-blind, placebo-controlled study of celecoxib, cyclooxygenase-2 inhibitor, in family adenomatous polyposis. *N Engl J Med* 2000; **26**: 1946–52.

18. *Anthony T, Rodriguez-Bigas M, Weber TK et al, Desmoid tumors. *J Am Coll Surg* 1996; **182**: 369–77.

19. *Jass JR, Williams CB, Bussey HJR et al, Juvenile polyposis – a precancerous condition. *Histopathology* 1988; **13**: 619–30.

20. Whitelaw SC, Murday VA, Tomlinson IPM et al, Clinical and molecular features of the hereditary mixed polyposis syndrome. *Gastroenterology* 1997; **112**: 327–34.

21. Desai DC, Neale KF, Talbot IC et al, Juvenile polyposis (Review). *Br J Surg* 1995; **82**: 14–17.

22. Houlston R, Bevan S, Williams A et al, Mutations in DPC4 (SMAD4) cause juvenile polyposis syndrome, but only account for minority of cases. *Hum Mol Genet* 1998; **7**: 1907–12.

23. Scott-Conner CEH, Hausmann M, Hall TJ et al, Familial juvenile polyposis: patterns of recurrence and implications for surgical management. *J Am Coll Surg* 1995; **181**: 407–13.

24. Rodriguez-Bigas MA, Penetrante RB, Herrera L et al, Intraoperative small bowel enteroscopy in familial adenomatous and familial juvenile polyposis. *Gastrointest Endosc* 1995; **42**: 560–4.

25. Hemminki A, The molecular basis and clinical aspects of Peutz–Jeghers syndrome (Review). *Cell Mol Life Sci* 1999; **55**: 735–50.

26. *Spigelman AD, Murday V, Phillips RKS, Cancer and the Peutz–Jeghers syndrome. *Gut* 1989; **30**: 1588–90.

27. Jiang C-Y, Esufali S, Berk T et al, *STK11/LKB1* germline mutations are not identified in most Peutz–Jeghers syndrome patients. *Clin Genet* 1999; **56**: 136–41.

28. *Lynch PM, Clinical challenges in management of familial adenomatous polyposis and hereditary non-polyposis colorectal cancer. *Cancer* 1999; **86**(Suppl): 2533–9.

29. Bapat BV, Madlensky L, Temple LKF et al, Family history characteristics, tumor microsatellite instability and germline *MSH2* and *MLH1* mutations in hereditary colorectal cancer. *Hum Genet* 1999; **104**: 167–76.

30. Vasen HFA, Wijnen JT, Menko FH et al, Cancer risk in families with hereditary nonpolyposis colorectal cancer diagnosed by mutation analysis. *Gastroenterology* 1996; **110**: 1020–7.

31. *Ponz de Leon M, Sassatelli R, Benatti P et al, Identificaton of hereditary nonpolyposis colorectal cancer in the general population. The 6-year experience of a population-based registry. *Cancer* 1993; **71**: 3493–501.

32. Thibodeau SN, French AM, Roche PC et al, Altered expression of hMSSH2 and hMLH1 in tumors with microsatellite instability and genetic alterations in mismatch repair genes. *Cancer Res* 1996; **56**: 4836–40.

33. *Burke W, Petersen G, Lynch P et al, Recommendations for follow-up care of individuals with an inherited predisposition to cancer. 1. Hereditary nonpolyposis colon cancer. *JAMA* 1997; **277**: 915–19.

34. *Vasen HFA, van Ballegooijen M, Buskens E et al. A cost-effectiveness analysis of colorectal screening of hereditary nonpolyposis colorectal carcinoma gene carriers. *Cancer* 1998; **82**: 1632–7.

35. Rodriguez-Bigas MA, Vasen HFA, Pekka-Mecklin J et al, Rectal cancer risk in hereditary nonpolyposis colorectal cancer after abdominal colectomy. *Ann Surg* 1997; **225**: 202–7.

36. Jarvinen HJ, Aarnio M, Mustonen H et al, Controlled 15-year trial on screening for colorectal cancer in families with hereditary non-polyposis colorectal cancer. *Gastroenterology* 2000; **118**: 829–34.

37. Sinicrope FAA, Lemoine M, Xi L et al, Reduced expression of cyclooxygenase 2 proteins in hereditary nonpolyposis colorectal cancers relative to sporadic cancers. *Gastroenterology* 1999; **117**: 350–8.

38. Carethers JM, Chauhan DP, Fink D et al, Mismatch repair proficiency and in vitro response to 5-fluorouracil. *Gastroenterology* 1999; **117**: 123–31.

39. Watson P, Lin KM, Rodriguez-Bigas M et al, Colorectal carcinoma survival among hereditary nonpolyposis colorectal carcinoma family members. *Cancer* 1998; **83**: 259–66.

40. *Rozen P, Shomrat R, Strul H et al, Prevalence of the I1307K *APC* gene variant in Israeli Jews of differing ethnic origin and risk for colorectal cancer. *Gastroenterology* 1999; **116**: 54–7.

41. St. John JB, McDermott FT, Hopper JL et al, Cancer risk in relatives of patients with common colorectal cancer. *Ann Intern Med* 1993; **118**: 785–90.

42. Fuchs CS, Giovannucci EL, Colditz GA et al, A prospective study of family history and the risk of colorectal cancer. *N Engl J Med* 1994; **331**: 1669–74.

43. *Winawer SJ, Zauber AG, Gerdes H et al, Risk of colorectal cancer in the families of patients with adenomatous polyps. *N Engl J Med* 1996; **334**: 82–7.

44. *Offit K, Brown K, Quantitating familial cancer risk: a resource for clinical oncologists. *J Clin Oncol* 1994; **12**: 1724–36.

45. Ulrich CM, Kampman E, Bigler J et al, Colorectal adenomas and the C677T *MTHFR* polymorphism: evidence for gene-environmental interaction? *Cancer Epidemiol Biomark Prev* 1999; **8**: 659–68.

46. Marchand LL, Wilkens LR, Hankin JH et al, Independent and joint effects of family history and lifestyle on colorectal cancer risk: implications for prevention. *Cancer Epidemiol Biomark Prev* 1999; **8**: 45–51.

47. Chapman PD, Burn J, Genetic predictive testing for bowel cancer predisposition: the impact on the individual. *Cytogenet Cell Genet* 1999; **86**: 118–24.

48. *Lynch HT, Watson P, Shaw TG et al, Clinical impact of molecular genetic diagnosis, genetic counseling, and management of hereditary cancer. Part I: Studies of cancer in families. *Cancer* 1999; **86**: 2449–56.

49. Lynch HT, Watson P, Shaw TG et al, Clinical impact of molecular genetic diagnosis, genetic counseling, and management of hereditary cancer. Part II: Hereditary nonpolyposis colorectal carcinoma as a model. *Cancer* 1999; **86**: 2457–63.

50. Kodish ED, Testing children for cancer genes: the rule of earliest onset. *J Pediatr* 1999; **135**: 390–5.

51. Vernon SW, Gritz ER, Peterson SK et al, Intention to learn results of genetic testing for hereditary colon cancer. *Cancer Epidemiol Biomark Prev* 1999; **8**: 353–60.

52. Wilcke JTR, Seersholm N, Kok-Jensen A et al, Transmitting genetic risk information in families: attitudes about disclosing the identity of relatives. *Am J Hum Genet* 1999; **65**: 902–9.

53. McEwen JE, McCarty K, Reilly PR, A survey of medical directors of life insurance companies concerning use of genetic information. *Am J Hum Genet* 1993; **53**: 33–45.

54. Rodriguez-Bigas M, Vasen HFA, O'Malley L et al, Health, life and disability insurance and hereditary nonpolyposis colorectal cancer. *Am J Hum Genet* 1998; **62**: 736–7.

55. Lynch PM, Jurisprudential considerations in the evaluation and screening of high-risk patients. In: *Secondary Prevention of Colorectal Cancer* (Rozen P, Winawer SJ, eds). Basel: Karger, 1986: 55–63.

56. *Lynch HT, Paulson J, Severin M et al, Failure to diagnose hereditary colorectal cancer and its medicolegal implications. A hereditary nonpolyposis colorectal cancer case. *Dis Colon Rectum* 1999; **42**: 31–5.

7 How should we follow up colorectal premalignant conditions?

Bernard Levin, Paul Rozen, Graeme P Young

Introduction

It is important to define with some precision the appropriate follow-up of patients at increased risk who have premalignant lesions of the colon and rectum. Such follow-up principally involves colonoscopic surveillance. While it is critical to detect neoplastic lesions at an early, pre-invasive stage, cost containment is another goal of a defined policy because of the expense of such surveillance. This chapter will focus on a discussion of follow-up after removal of colorectal adenomas, and on endoscopic surveillance of patients with chronic inflammatory bowel disease and of women with a history of breast or gynecological cancer.

Follow-up after removal of colorectal adenomas

Classification of large-bowel polyps

For a description of how polyps are classified and their malignant potential, see Table 7.1 and Figure 7.1 (see also Chapter 6, Figure 6.2). By definition, adenomatous epithelium is neoplastic, and all adenomas exhibit some degree of dysplasia. Dysplasia may be classified as mild (low grade), moderate, or severe (high grade). The degree of cytologic atypia and glandular architectural distortion determines the grade of dysplasia. At clinical discovery, approximately 5% of adenomas contain high-grade dysplasia and 2.5% contain invasive cancer.[1,2] The correct term for a lesion with invasive cancer is an adenoma-containing adenocarcinoma.[2] Villous histology, severe dysplasia, and size 1 cm or more are all associated with an increased risk of cancer within the adenoma, and are sometimes referred to as 'advanced pathology'[3] (Table 7.2).

Flat adenomas

Recent reports, particularly from Japan, have demonstrated that 'flat adenomas' are more likely to contain carcinoma or severe dysplasia than sessile adenomas of a similar size.[4] Flat lesions can be defined endoscopically

Table 7.1 Classification of large-bowel non-cancerous polypoid lesions and their relative malignant potential

Mucosal lesion	Malignant potential
Neoplasia[a]	
Tubular adenoma	+
Tubular villous adenoma	+ +
Villous adenoma	+ + +
Non-neoplastic	
Hyperplastic polyp	–
Serrated adenoma[b]	+
(mixed hyperplastic and	
adenomatous polyp)	
Juvenile polyp (polyposis)[b]	– / + + +
Peutz–Jeghers polyps[b]	– / +
Inflammatory polyp	–
Submucosal lesion	
Lipoma	–
Carcinoid	– / +
Colitis cystic profunda	–

[a] The larger the adenoma, the more the villous elements, the greater the risk for cancer.
[b] The greater the number of adenomatous elements occurring in this non-neoplastic polyp, the greater the risk for cancer. See also Chapter 6.

and histologically. Histologically, the dysplastic tissue does not protrude above the mucosal surface, and the dysplastic tissue is no more than twice the thickness of the mucosa (Figure 7.2). Endoscopically, these lesions are less than 1 cm in diameter, and have a non-exophytic flat-topped shape, sometimes with a central red-colored depression.

These flat lesions have been reported from European countries, and in a recent British series of asymptomatic persons undergoing flexible sigmoidoscopy, the incidence was 1 in 1000 examinations.[5] In the USA, current evidence suggests that clinically important flat lesions, with a high malignant potential, are unlikely to be frequently

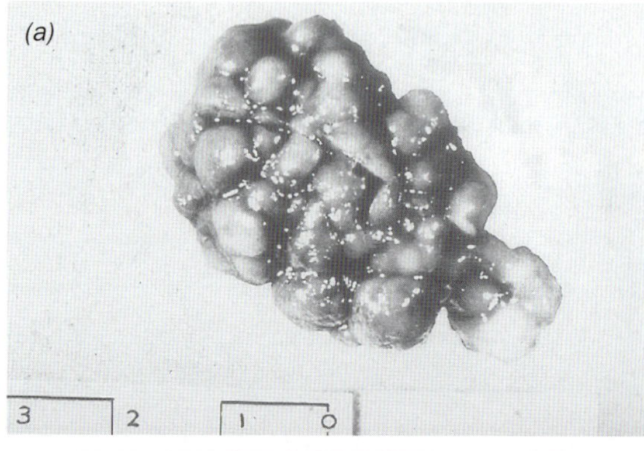
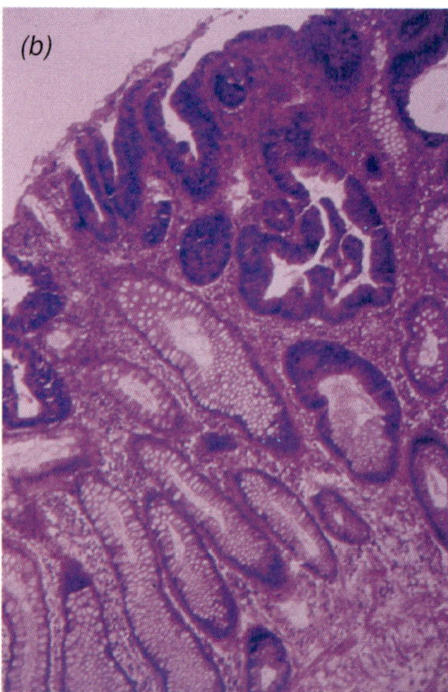
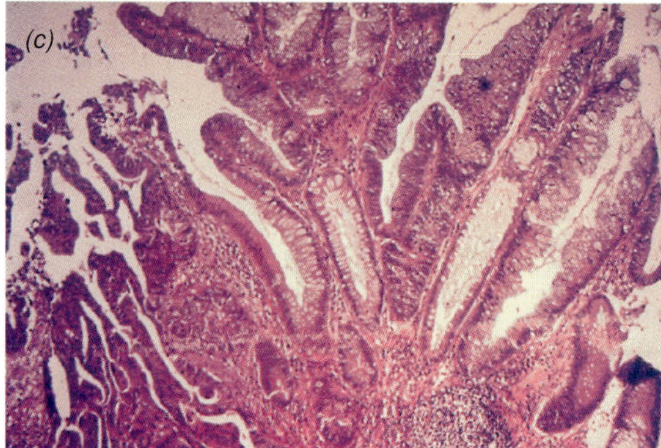
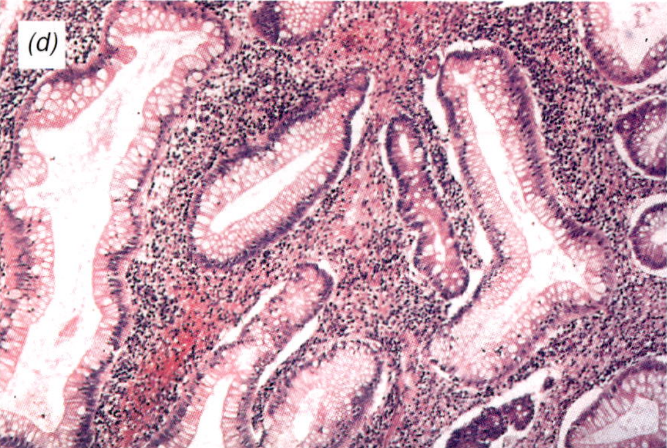

Figure 7.1 (a) A large adenomatous polyp removed at colonoscopy. (b) Histological section demonstrated a tubular adenoma with an area of localized high-grade dysplasia. Note the dark-staining crowded nuclei in the superficial portion of the section. (c) A villous adenoma. Note the frond-like appearance of the mucosa on the right side of the section, and the area of high-grade dysplasia with dark staining and crowded and disorganized nuclei on the left side of the section. (d) Polyp from a patient with familial juvenile polyposis. The polyp demonstrates dilated glands lined by normal-appearing epithelium with inflammatory cells densely packed in the stroma, typical of a juvenile polyp. However, some of the glands are lined by dark oval nuclei typical of adenomatous changes.

Table 7.2 High-grade dysplasia found in adenomas removed by colonoscopy, by size and histology (n = 3371)[a]

Histology	Size (cm)		
	<0.5	0.6–1.0	>1.0
Tubular	0.7%	2.7%	7.4%
Tubulovillous	14.7%	19.6%	31.7%
Villous	20.0%	17.6%	35.0%

[a] Adapted from reference 3.

overlooked.[6] For example, in the National Polyp Study, the incidence of diminutive adenomas was 0.9%, and those who had undergone polypectomy had a low risk of subsequent colorectal cancer.[7] The different incidence, size, and numbers of adenomas found in some other countries, such as Japan and Israel, probably reflect the effects of different diets, lifestyle, and genetic pathways to carcinogenesis.

Incidence

The incidence of colonic adenomas increases with age in countries with a high or intermediate risk for colorectal cancer. At autopsy, adenomas are found in 30–50% of individuals older than 60 years of age in the USA and other Western countries[8] (Table 7.3). In a recent study of over 3000 US Army veterans (96% men) whose mean age was 63 years, colonoscopic examination showed one or more neoplastic lesions in 38% of the patients, an adenoma with a diameter of at least 10 mm or a villous adenoma in 8%, an adenoma with high-grade dysplasia in 2%, and invasive

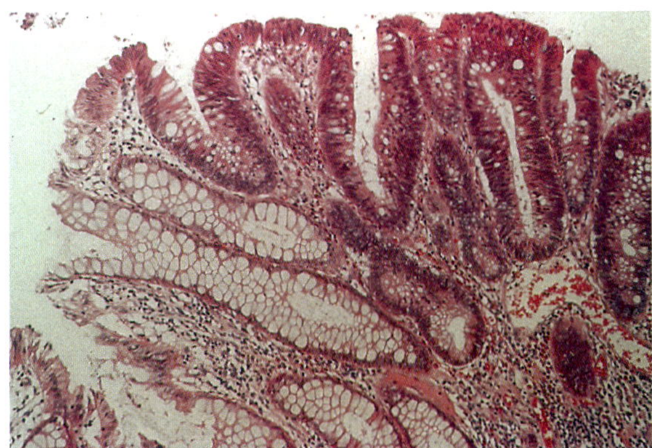

Figure 7.2 *Photomicrograph of a 'flat' adenoma, which appears to be in the same plane as the surrounding mucosa.*

Table 7.3 *Prevalence of adenomas in selected autopsy studies*[a]

Study location	Years	Prevalence (%)	
		Men	**Women**
USA			
Hawaii	1969–1984	64	57
New Orleans	1970–1975	36	20
New York	1960	40	37
Europe			
Oslo, Norway	1974–1976	40	33
Liverpool, UK		37	29
Asia			
Akita, Japan	1970–1973	38	24
Hong Kong	1985	19	34
South America			
Cali, Colombia		6.0	5.0

[a] Modified from reference 8 with permission.

cancer in 1%.[9] In Hawaii, the incidence of colorectal cancer among people of Japanese descent is extremely high, and parallels their high prevalence rate of adenomas, which is higher than that found in Japanese residents in Japan. In contrast, however, in a multicenter endoscopic screening study of 3000 average-risk persons in Israel (which has a high incidence of colorectal cancer), adenomas were found in only about 2%, and only half were larger than 0.5 cm.[10] Similarly, only a 5% prevalence of adenomas was found at autopsy studies in Cali, Colombia (Table 7.3). Because of the high prevalence of adenomas in some Western countries, the management of adenomas, and especially post-polypectomy surveillance, has substantial economic implications. Fortunately, there is considerable experience and information available upon which to base recommendations, including the results of several large studies such as the US National Polyp Study[11] discussed below.

Clinical significance of distal adenomas

In a British study, 1618 patients were treated for rectosigmoid adenomas using rigid sigmoidoscopy.[12] The study was done in the pre-colonoscopy era. These patients were not initially followed up, and the study retrospectively assessed their long-term risk of developing colorectal cancer. The risk of subsequent colon cancer was increased 1.7-fold when a single adenoma was detected and 4.8-fold if multiple adenomas were present, but was not increased when only a single small (1 cm or less) tubular adenoma was detected. This has led to a large-scale randomized trial of flexible sigmoidoscopy in the UK to evaluate the cancer-preventive usefulness of removing small rectosigmoid adenomas.

Recently, investigators determined the risk of having an advanced proximal neoplasm, among persons with or without distal neoplastic polyps.[13] The prevalence of advanced proximal neoplasm among patients with no distal adenomas was 1.5%. Among patients with distal tubular adenomas, and those with advanced distal polyps, the prevalences of advanced proximal neoplasms were 7.1% and 11.5% respectively. Age over 50 years and male sex increased the risk of having an advanced proximal neoplasm 3.5-fold. Based on these findings and other data,[14] at present, colonoscopy is advised for patients with a distal adenoma of any size found at flexible sigmoidoscopy.

Risk for cancer

Important in the development of a strategy for surveillance is an understanding of the biology of adenomas. Few adenomatous polyps progress to cancer; the rate is estimated at about 2.5 polyps per 1000 per year.[3] The transformation seems to occur over many years, and estimates are based on largely indirect evidence. These include observations on biopsied polyps that are not removed and their transformation to cancer over a period of 10–15 years. Another line of evidence derives from data on the mean age of people with early adenomatous polyps and those with colorectal cancer. The average age difference was 18 years.

Clinical effectiveness of polypectomy

Encouraging evidence related to the effectiveness of post-polypectomy colonoscopic surveillance derives from the US National Polyp Study, where a cohort of 1418 patients had undergone complete colonoscopy and removal of one or more adenomatous polyps from the colon.[15] These individuals were followed for an average of 5.9 years per patient. After adjusting for adenoma size, age, and sex, the rates of cancer were 76–90% lower than expected in comparison with three reference groups (Figure 7.3). However, this was not a randomized clinical trial.

Post-polypectomy surveillance

The investigators in the National Polyp Study determined the optimal frequency of surveillance in patients who had undergone prior polypectomy and who were randomized to undergo surveillance colonoscopy either at 1 and 3 years or only 3 years after polypectomy.[15] The two groups showed no difference in the proportion of detection of adenomatous polyps with advanced pathology (3.3% in both groups; 95% confidence interval (CI) 0.8–5.3%). These data suggest that the first follow-up colonoscopic examination after polypectomy can be deferred for 3 years. A longer follow-up interval of 6 years has been proposed for subjects other than those who have three or more adenomas at initial colonoscopy or who are 60 years of age or over and have a first-degree relative with colorectal cancer. Similar conclusions have been reached by other investigators.[16]

The following management guidelines have been developed by the National Health and Medical Research Council of Australia.[17] Colonoscopic surveillance should be implemented:

(1) at three months following piecemeal removal, or excision of a malignant adenoma, or a large adenoma that may have been excised incompletely;
(2) within a year following incomplete or possibly inadequate examination – for example in a subject with multiple adenomas;
(3) at 3 years for subjects with high-grade dysplasia, villous changes in adenomas, or three or more adenomas, or in those aged 60 years or older and who have a first-degree relative with colorectal cancer;
(4) at 4–6 years in subjects without the preceding risk factors.

These recommendations are similar to those suggested by a consortium of US gastroenterology societies under the auspices of the Agency for Health Care Policy and Research of the USA.[11]

Future developments

For individuals who are prone to adenoma recurrence, chemopreventive measures may be useful to reduce the risk of recurrence. Examples of such agents include folic acid, aspirin, the bile salt ursodiol, and non-steroidal anti-inflammatory drugs (NSAIDs) including exisulind (sulindac

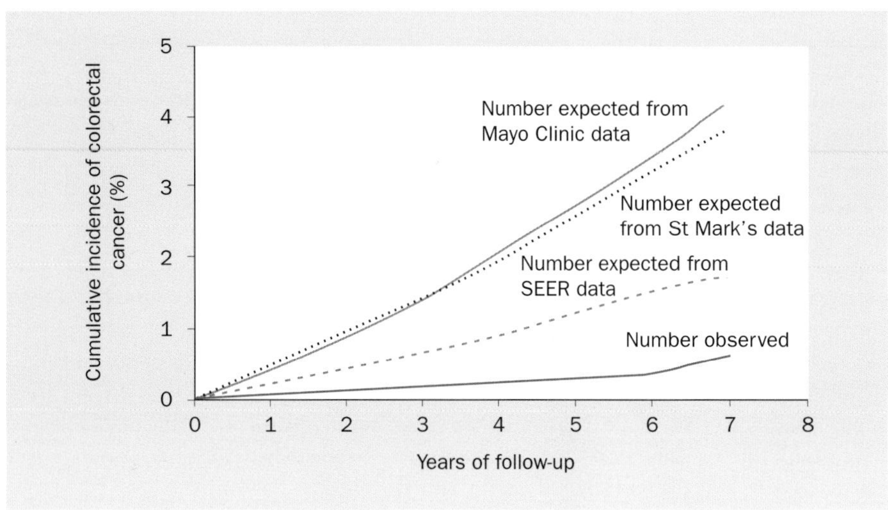

Figure 7.3 *Cumulative observed incidence of colorectal cancer in the US National Polyp Study cohort was significantly less than that estimated to occur in two reference populations. Reproduced with permission from Winawer SJ et al, N Engl J Med 1993; 328: 901–6.[15] ©1993 Massachusetts Medical Society. All rights reserved.*

sulfone) and cyclooxygenase-2 (COX-2) inhibitors such as celecoxib and rofecoxib.[18] Clinical trials of these compounds are in progress in Europe, Australia, Israel, and North and South America. It is premature to recommend any specific chemopreventive intervention at this time (see also Chapter 5).

Chronic inflammatory bowel disease

Introduction

Among all patients diagnosed with a large-bowel carcinoma, about 1% give an antecedent history of ulcerative colitis or Crohn's disease. The management of those at risk poses a challenge for both patient and physician. Specific guidelines for Crohn's disease have not been established, so this discussion will focus predominantly on ulcerative colitis.

Ulcerative colitis
Clinical features

In a patient with longstanding ulcerative colitis, the patient or physician may attribute symptoms such as rectal bleeding, abdominal cramping or diarrhea to colitis and the diagnosis of carcinoma may be missed until far advanced.

Risk factors for neoplasia

The two best-established risk factors for developing colorectal cancer in ulcerative colitis are anatomical extent of colonic involvement and duration of disease. Patients with extensive colitis (disease proximal to the splenic flexure) are at greatest risk, whereas those who have only proctitis do not have an increased risk of cancer.[19] Those with left-sided disease are also at increased risk, and surveillance is advised after 12 years of disease.[20]

Colorectal cancer is rare when the duration of pancolitis is less than 8 years. The risk begins to rise above that of the general population after about 8–10 years of the disease. Although earlier retrospective reports from specialty referral centers had reported higher cancer rates, current estimates from population-based studies indicate that the cumulative incidence ranges between 5% and 10% after 20 years' disease duration and between 12% and 20% after 30 years.[19] Contrary to earlier views, age at onset does not seem to be an independent risk factor,[20,21] but young patients are more likely to have pancolitis and, over the ensuing years, be more susceptible to cancer than those with more limited disease.

The use of sulfasalazine in the management of chronic ulcerative colitis has been associated with folate deficiency. Clinical studies have suggested an association between folate deficiency and colorectal dysplasia in these patients.[22] Folate supplementation (400 µg/day) seems to be an innocuous and possibly helpful intervention, but, so far, is of unproven value.

Clinicopathological features of neoplasia

The macroscopic appearances are heterogeneous, and include strictures, nodules, plaques, and irregular polypoid masses.[19] Some cancers arise in totally flat mucosa, and may be detected only by chance. Fixed colonic strictures should be regarded with suspicion, and have been reported to harbor cancer in 24–40% of cases (Figure 7.4). Multiple synchronous colorectal cancers occur much more frequently in inflammatory bowel disease than in the general population.[19] Microscopically, mucinous adenocarcinomas are twice as common in ulcerative colitis as compared with sporadic cancers.

Pathogenesis of cancer in ulcerative colitis

Although there is little difference between the overall and stage-adjusted survival rates of cancer in chronic ulcerative colitis or in the general population, the early diagnosis of cancer is an important goal. Both sporadic colorectal cancer and colitis-associated large-bowel cancer arise from dysplastic precursors. Sporadic colorectal cancer usually arises from an adenomatous polyp, whereas colitis-associated cancer typically arises from flat dysplasia or a dysplasia-associated lesion or mass (DALM). Dysplasia is defined as an unequivocal neoplastic alteration of the large-bowel epithelium confined within the basement membrane in which it arises; regenerative and reactive changes resulting from inflammation are excluded. The

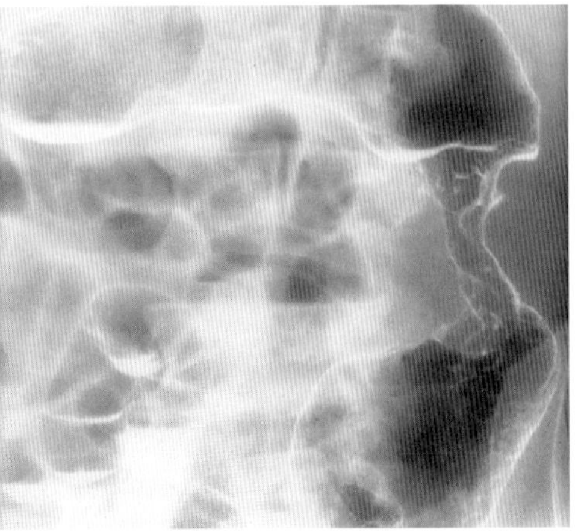

Figure 7.4 *Radiograph demonstrating a colonic stricture and synchronous cancers in a patient with ulcerative colitis. Note the lack of haustra, which is typical of longstanding and extensive colitis.*

nomenclature and criteria for assessment of dysplasia have been standardized (Table 7.4).[23] Examples of dysplastic changes are illustrated in Figure 7.5.

Patient management

The management possibilities for patients at increased risk for colorectal cancer include prophylactic proctocolectomy or periodic endoscopic surveillance. An onset of total ulcerative colitis in childhood or adolescence may convey a high enough risk to warrant prophylactic surgery. The patient who faces a lifelong program of colonoscopic surveillance may be better served by a prophylactic colectomy. Moreover, owing to advances in surgical technique, a permanent stoma can be avoided by forming an ileoanal anastomosis using a pouch of small intestine as reservoir. The decision to recommend surgical removal of the large bowel must be based on individual considerations, including intractability of symptoms, ease of access to continued medical care including regular colonoscopic surveillance, psychological factors, age, and good anal sphincter function. Particularly in young patients, the quality of life after proctocolectomy is extremely good, even though attacks of inflammation are not uncommon in the ileal pouch ('pouchitis'). For optimal results, surgical management should be performed by an experienced colorectal surgical team. In some cases, the surgeon and older patients may choose an ileorectal anastomosis if the rectal inflammation is in remission. If so, then this demands careful follow-up surveillance (see below).

Surveillance in practice

The rationale for cancer surveillance in ulcerative colitis is based on the assumption that dysplasia is a reliable marker for pre-neoplasia or cancer and that surveillance detects cancer at an earlier stage, hence improving survival. The aim of surveillance is to intervene before the development of cancer. Cancer surveillance is a continuous process of clinical evaluation and investigation.[24,25] Colonoscopy is used initially during the early years of the disease to determine the extent of colonic involvement; subsequently annual surveillance colonoscopies are performed in those with 8–10 years of symptoms and extensive colitis (involvement extending to the hepatic flexure). For those with colitis confined to the left side of the colon, surveillance should begin after 12 years of symptoms. Multiple biopsies are obtained at 10–12 cm intervals throughout the colon, including the cecum, ascending colon, hepatic flexure, transverse colon, splenic flexure, descending colon, sigmoid, and rectum. Approximately 30–35 biopsies are obtained during this procedure. At least two-thirds of neoplasms or dysplastic changes occur in the rectosigmoid. For this reason, if annual colonoscopy is difficult to arrange or is unacceptable to the patient, then a compromise in which examination by flexible sigmoidoscopy replaces colonoscopy every second year may be preferable to infrequent surveillance.[25] The histological findings and recommended clinical actions are summarized in Table 7.4.

A management algorithm is presented in Figure 7.6. If no dysplastic changes are found, surveillance is repeated at 1- to 2-year intervals. In the presence of indefinite

Table 7.4 *Biopsy classification of dysplasia in inflammatory bowel disease and recommended clinical action in the course of endoscopic surveillance*

Pathological findings[a]	Recommended clinical action
● Negative for dysplasia	
Normal mucosa	Continue periodic surveillance
Inactive colitis	Continue periodic surveillance
Active colitis	Treat colitis
● Indefinite for dysplasia	Repeat surveillance in 6 months
● Positive for dysplasia	
Low-grade dysplasia	Proctocolectomy, or repeat biopsies in 3–4 months, colectomy if confirmed
High-grade dysplasia	Proctocolectomy
● Sessile lesion (dysplasia-associated mass)	Proctocolectomy
● Polypoid adenomas in non-dysplastic epithelium	Colonoscopic polypectomy

[a] Adapted from reference 23.

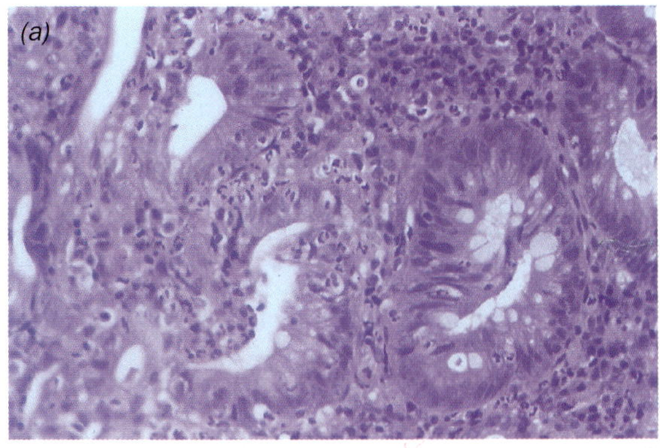

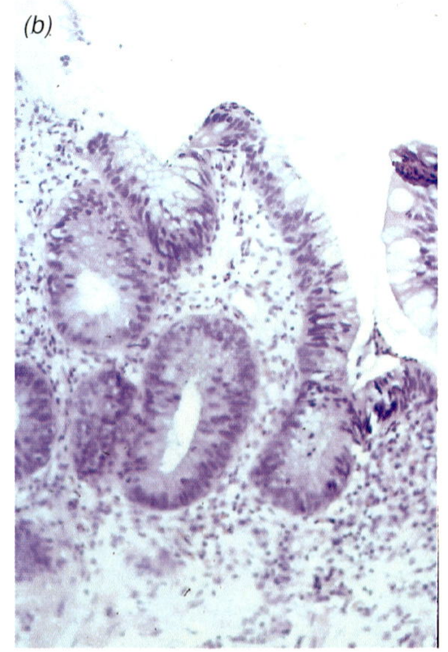

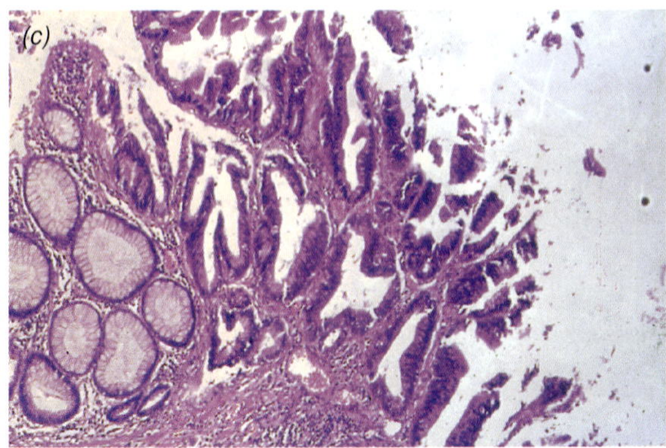

Figure 7.5 *Photomicrographs of dysplastic changes occurring in chronic ulcerative colitis.*
(a) A screening biopsy taken at random from a patient with longstanding, extensive, and mildly active ulcerative colitis. The crypts are distorted and the epithelial cells have hyperchromatic stratified nuclei. There is dense stromal inflammation, which enters the glands (cryptitis). This regenerative atypia cannot be easily differentiated from low-grade dysplasia; thus, this case is classified as indeterminate dysplasia, probably negative.
(b) A screening biopsy taken from the rectum of a patient with longstanding, extensive, but quiescent ulcerative colitis. The crypts' lining cells have hyperchromatic stratified nuclei, which are also seen in the surface epithelial cells. There is relatively little stromal inflammation. This was classified as low-grade dysplasia. Endoscopy repeated a few months later demonstrated a small nodular mass in the rectum, which on repeated biopsies demonstrated high-grade dysplasia. Colectomy was performed, and the final diagnosis was adenocarcinoma that did not invade through the entire rectal wall.
(c) Screening biopsy from a patient with longstanding, extensive ulcerative colitis in clinical remission. A small, elevated irregular lesion was identified at endoscopy. On the left side of the figure, the crypts are slightly distorted and are lined with dark-staining basal nuclei, compatible with ulcerative colitis in remission. On the right side, there are distorted glands with a villiform appearance, and the dark-staining nuclei are stratified, compatible with high-grade dysplasia.

dysplasia, colonoscopy should be repeated in 6 months. High-grade dysplasia (HGD), whether it occurs in a mass lesion or in flat mucosa, is considered an indication for colectomy. The cancer risk is also high enough to warrant colectomy if low-grade dysplasia (LGD) is found in a mass lesion. When LGD is detected in flat mucosa, the high risk of progression to HGD or cancer warrants a policy of early colectomy. Some recommend a repeat colonoscopy 3–6 months later to confirm the presence of LGD before proceeding with removal of the colon. If the presence of LGD is not confirmed, yearly surveillance is continued. The key to all colonoscopic surveillance is reliance on an expert gastrointestinal pathologist for interpretation of the mucosal biopsies and correlation with clinical findings. This is particularly crucial when making decisions about the management of HGD or LGD.

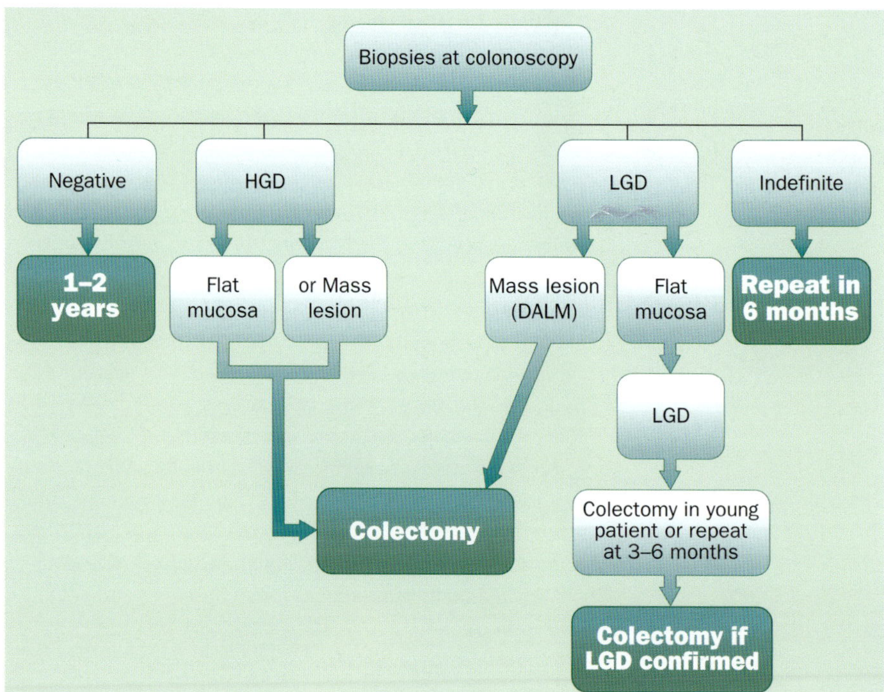

Figure 7.6 *Patient management algorithm in chronic ulcerative colitis surveillance. HGD, high-grade dysplasia; LGD, low-grade dysplasia; DALM, dysplasia-associated lesion or mass.*

Adenomas in the ulcerative colitis patient

In patients who do not have pancolitis, an adenoma may arise on normal colonic mucosa within the proximal colon. Such adenomas may be either pedunculated or sessile, and should be managed as they would in a patient without colitis. If a sessile adenoma arises within bowel involved by the colitic process, it cannot reliably be differentiated from a dysplastic mass, and a colectomy may be the most prudent clinical action. When a pedunculated adenoma arises in a colon involved by colitis, the adjacent and remote mucosa should be sampled during colonoscopic polypectomy. If there is no evidence of dysplasia beyond the adenoma, no further action is needed. If dysplasia is present elsewhere, a colectomy is recommended. Recently, a more conservative approach has been suggested for the management of sporadic adenoma-like dysplastic lesions occurring in ulcerative colitis patients, but this remains highly controversial.[26]

Patients with ileorectal anastomosis

Patients with an ileorectal anastomosis and a history of chronic ulcerative colitis remain at risk for the development of rectal cancer. For this reason, the procedure has fallen out of favor. In the presence of a retained rectal segment, periodic endoscopic surveillance with multiple biopsies should be performed according to the previous guidelines.

Sclerosing cholangitis and cholangiocarcinoma

Primary sclerosing cholangitis has been reported to occur in both ulcerative colitis and Crohn's disease. Patients with ulcerative colitis and sclerosing cholangitis have an increased risk of developing colorectal cancer and also a risk of developing cholangiocarcinoma in either the extra-hepatic or intrahepatic biliary tract. The disease may be clinically silent for a lengthy period, with the gradual onset of non-specific symptoms and/or a rising serum alkaline phosphatase found incidentally. Endoscopic retrograde cholangiography (ERCP) is useful for establishing a diagnosis. Magnetic resonance cholangio-pancreatography is likely to be used with increasing frequency, particularly when ERCP is not successful.

Effectiveness of surveillance

Randomized controlled trials on the effectiveness of surveillance in patients with longstanding ulcerative colitis have not been conducted. A summary of prospective cohort studies from both the USA and Europe suggests that the percentage of advanced colon cancers with bad outcome is reduced by surveillance to 35%.[24,25] This can be compared with 60% of patients diagnosed with stage 3 and 4 colon cancer in series of ulcerative colitis patients from outside of surveillance programs. The finding of stage 3 or stage 4 cancer in patients enrolled in a surveillance program constitutes a failure of the program.[25]

Future developments

More accurate and better methods of surveillance are needed. Based on recent findings, genomic instability and microsatellite instability occur early on in the course of dysplasia development, and may afford an opportunity for earlier diagnosis on biopsy and differentiation from inflammatory and adenomatous tissue (see Chapter 3).[27,28] The potential role of molecular-marker detection in the stool is under investigation in the non-colitic population and may be applicable in the future to surveillance.[29] Laser-induced fluorescence using δ-aminolevulinic acid sensitization can discriminate in vivo between normal tissue and adenomatous polyps.[30] It remains to be seen whether this technique can be applied to surveillance in ulcerative colitis or Crohn's disease.

Crohn's disease

Cancer of the large bowel

There is a significantly increased incidence of colorectal cancer in patients with extensive colonic involvement. Those with longstanding anorectal involvement also appear to be at significantly increased risk of developing anal or rectal malignancies. Although dysplasia is well recognized, surveillance in patients with Crohn's disease of the large bowel may be technically difficult because of the presence of strictures and fistulous disease.[25] For these reasons, there are no established surveillance protocols in this disease other than to emphasize heightened clinical awareness.

Cancer of the small bowel

Small-bowel cancer in the general population is extremely rare, but is more common in patients with Crohn's disease of the small bowel, particularly in association with fistulous disease and bypassed loops of bowel. There is a long latency period between disease onset and occurrence of cancer (with a mean of 18 years). In Crohn's disease, two-thirds of cancers occur in the ileum, whereas in the general population small-bowel tumors are more evenly distributed throughout the small intestine. Again, clinical awareness is the only surveillance method available to detect malignant change.

Women with breast and gynecological cancer

Meta-analyses of follow-up studies have suggested that women with prior ovarian or endometrial cancer have an increased relative risk of subsequent colorectal cancer. This risk is greater than the relative risk of 1.1 for colorectal cancer in women with prior breast cancer.[31,32] There is no increased risk of colorectal cancer in women with cervical cancer.[33] Analysis of SEER (Surveillance, Epidemiology and End Results Program, USA) data has demonstrated that the increased risk of colorectal cancer is confined to women diagnosed with endometrial cancer before age 50 years or ovarian cancer before age 65 years.[33] The respective relative risks are as follows: for those with ovarian cancer before age 50 years, 3.67 (95% CI 2.74 – 4.88); for those with ovarian cancer above age 50 years, 1.52 (95% CI 1.25–1.83); and for those with endometrial cancer before age 50 years, 3.9 (95% CI 2.73–4.17). In approaching risk assessment in women with prior endometrial or ovarian cancer, a detailed family history should be obtained to identify kindreds with an established genetic syndrome such as hereditary non-polyposis colorectal cancer (HNPCC), and appropriate screening measures can then be implemented (see Chapter 6).[34] If the woman was diagnosed with endometrial cancer at age less than 50 years or ovarian cancer at less than 64 years and the family history does not meet or approach the criteria for HNPCC, then a colonoscopy at 3- to 5-year intervals is advised. The basis for this recommendation is that the relative risk of colorectal cancer in such patients is comparable to the risk in first-degree relatives of patients diagnosed with colorectal cancer or with adenomas at a young age.[35]

For patients diagnosed with ovarian cancer over the age of 64 years and endometrial cancer after age 50 years, average-risk screening approaches are adequate.

Future developments

As risk models are developed, it is likely that surveillance recommendations will be increasingly refined so that only the most cost-effective and beneficial approaches are selected.

References (*Reviews and general articles)

1. *Markowitz AJ, Winawer SJ, Screening and surveillance for colorectal cancer. *Semin Oncol* 1991; **26**: 485–98.

2. *Hamilton SR, Pathology and biology of colorectal neoplasia. In: *Prevention and Early Detection of Colorectal Cancer* (Young GP, Rozen P, Levin B, eds). London: Saunders, 1996: 3–21.

3. *O'Brien MJ, Winawer SJ, Zauber AG et al, The National Polyp Study: patient and polyp characteristics associated with high grade dysplasia in colorectal adenomas. *Gastroenterology* 1990; **98**: 371–9.

4. Mitooka H, Fujimora T, Maeda S, Minute flat depressed neoplastic lesions of the colon detected by contrast chromoscopy using an indigo carmine capsule. *Gastrointest Endosc* 1995; **41**: 453–9.

5. Hart AR, Kudo S, MacKay EH et al, Flat adenomas exist in asymptomatic people: important implications for colorectal cancer screening programmes. *Gut* 1998; **43**: 229–31.

6. Bond JH, Comment. *Gastrointest Endosc* 1999; **50**: 589–90.

7. *Winawer SJ, Zauber AG, Ho MN et al, Prevention of colorectal cancers by colonoscopic polypectomy. *N Engl J Med* 1993; **329**: 1977–81.

8. *Peipins LA, Sandler RS, Epidemiology of colorectal adenomas. *Epidemiol Rev* 1994; **16**: 273–97.

9. Lieberman DA, Weiss DG, Bond JH et al, Use of colonoscopy to screen asymptomatic adults for colorectal cancer. *N Engl J Med* 2000; **343**: 162–8.

10. Odes HS, Rozen P, Ron E et al, Screening for colorectal neoplasia: a multicenter study in Israel. *Isr J Med Sci* 1992; **28**(Suppl): 21–8.

11. *Winawer SJ, Fletcher RH, Miller L et al, Colorectal cancer screening clinical guidelines and rationale. *Gastroenterology* 1997; **112**: 594–642.

12. Atkin WS, Morson BC, Cuzick J, Longterm risk of colorectal cancer after excision of rectosigmoid adenomas. *N Engl J Med* 1992; **26**: 658–62.

13. Imperale TF, Wagner DR, Lin CY et al, Risk of advanced proximal neoplasms in asymptomatic adults according to the distal colorectal findings. *N Engl J Med* 2000; **343**: 169–74.

14. Rex DK, Chak A, Vasuveda R et al, Prospective determination of distal colon findings in average risk patients with proximal colon cancer. *Gastrointest Endosc* 1999; **49**: 727–30.

15. Winawer SJ, Zauber AG, O'Brien MJ et al, Randomized comparison of surveillance intervals after colonoscopic removal of newly diagnosed adenomatous polyps. *N Engl J Med* 1993; **328**: 901–6.

16. Noshiswani K, von Stolk R, Rybicki L et al, Adenoma size and number are predictive of adenoma recurrence. *Gastrointest Endosc* 2000; **51**: 433–7.

17. *National Health and Medical Research Council, Australia, *Clinical Practice Guidelines. The Prevention, Early Detection and Management of Colorectal Cancer.* Commonwealth of Australia, 1999, www.ausinfo.gov.au/general/gen_hottobouy.htm.

18. Steinbach G, Lynch PM, Phillips RKS et al, The effect of celecoxib, a cyclooxygenase-2 inhibitor, in familial adenomatous polyposis. *N Engl J Med* 2000; **342**: 1946–52.

19. Harpaz N, Talbot IC, Colorectal cancer in idiopathic inflammatory bowel disease. *Semin Diagn Pathol* 1996; **13**: 339–57.

20. Ekbom A, Helmick C, Zach M et al, Ulcerative colitis and colorectal cancer: a population-based study. *N Engl J Med* 1990; **323**: 1228–33.

21. Ahsgren L, Jonsson B, Sterling R et al, Prognosis after early onset of ulcerative colitis: a study from an unselected patient population. *Hepato Gastroenterol* 1993; **40**: 467–70.

22. Lashner BA, Provencher KS, Seidner DL et al, The effect of folic acid supplementation on the risk for cancer or dysplasia in ulcerative colitis. *Gastroenterology* 1997; **112**: 29–32.

23. Riddell RH, Goldman H, Ransohoff DF et al, Dysplasia in inflammatory bowel disease: standardized classification with provisional clinical applications. *Hum Pathol* 1983; **14**: 931–68.

24. Griffiths AM, Sherman PM, Colonoscopic surveillance for cancer in ulcerative colitis: a critical review. *J Pediatr Gastroenterol Nutr* 1997; **24**: 202–10.

25. *Lennard-Jones JE, Prevention of cancer mortality in inflammatory bowel disease. In: *Prevention and Early Detection of Colorectal Cancer* (Young GP, Rozen P, Levin B, eds). London: Saunders, 1996: 217–38.

26. Engelsgjerd M, Farraye FA, Odze RD, Polypectomy may be adequate treatment for adenoma-like dysplastic lesions in chronic ulcerative colitis. *Gastroenterology* 1999; **117**: 1288–4.

27. Willenbucher RF, Aust DE, Chang CG et al, Genomic instability is an early event during the progression pathway of ulcerative-colitis related neoplasia. *Am J Pathol* 1999; **154**: 1825–30.

28. Mueller E, Vieth M, Stolte M et al, The differentiation of true adenomas from colitis-associated dysplasia in ulcerative colitis: a comparative immunohistochemical study. *Hum Pathol* 1999; **30**: 898–905.

29. Jen J, Johnson C, Levin B, Molecular approaches for colorectal cancer screening. *Eur J Gastroenterol Hepatol* 1998; **10**: 213–17.

30. Eker C, Montan S, Jaramillo E et al, Clinical spectral characterization of colonic mucosal lesions using autofluorescence and delta amino levulinic acid sensitization. *Gut* 1999; **44**: 511–18.

31. Schoen RE, Weissfeld JL, Kuller LH, Are women with breast, endometrial or ovarian cancer at increased risk for colorectal cancer? *Am J Gastroenterol* 1994; **89**: 835–42.

32. Eisen GM, Sandler RS, Are women with breast cancer more likely to develop colorectal cancer? Critical review and meta-analyses. *J Clin Gastroenterol* 1994; **19**: 57–63.

33. Weinberg DS, Newtschaffer CJ, Tophan BA, Risk for colorectal cancer after gynecologic cancer. *Ann Intern Med* 1999; **131**: 189–93.

34. Rex D, Comment. *Am J Gastroenterol* 2000; **95**: 812–13.

35. St John DJB, McDermott FT, Hopper JL et al, Cancer risk in relatives of patients with common colorectal cancer. *Ann Intern Med* 1995; **118**: 785–90.

8 How should we screen for early colorectal neoplasia?

Graeme P Young, Paul Rozen, Bernard Levin

Introduction

The biology of colorectal cancer provides opportunities for preventive strategies based on the early detection of curable cancer or removable adenoma. The process of cancer development (as described in Chapter 3) consists of multiple steps; some events (especially polypoid adenomas and microscopic, or occult, bleeding) are recognizable clinically at premalignant stages. The process extends over a considerable period of time, possibly as long as 10 years in non-familial cancers. Figure 8.1 shows in diagrammatic form how various forms of tests can be applied to the stages of tumorigenesis.

From the perspective of healthcare policy, colorectal cancer meets the requirements of the World Health Organization (WHO) for suitability for screening.[1] Screening for colorectal cancer first became feasible when Greegor described the use of the fecal occult blood test (FOBT) for early detection.[2]

While countries such as Germany, Japan, Israel, and the USA have given conditional support to population screening,[3] some primary-care practitioners remain pessimistic about the ability of screening to reduce mortality in the USA[4] as well as in other Western countries such as Australia. In practice, the reasons that lead to a country providing population screening on an organized basis are somewhat different to those to be considered at the time of the highly personal doctor–patient interaction. With the former, issues relate to costs, resources, and health-funding models. Issues with the latter relate to duty of care and personal choice. As screening of healthy people is ultimately an important issue for the community as a

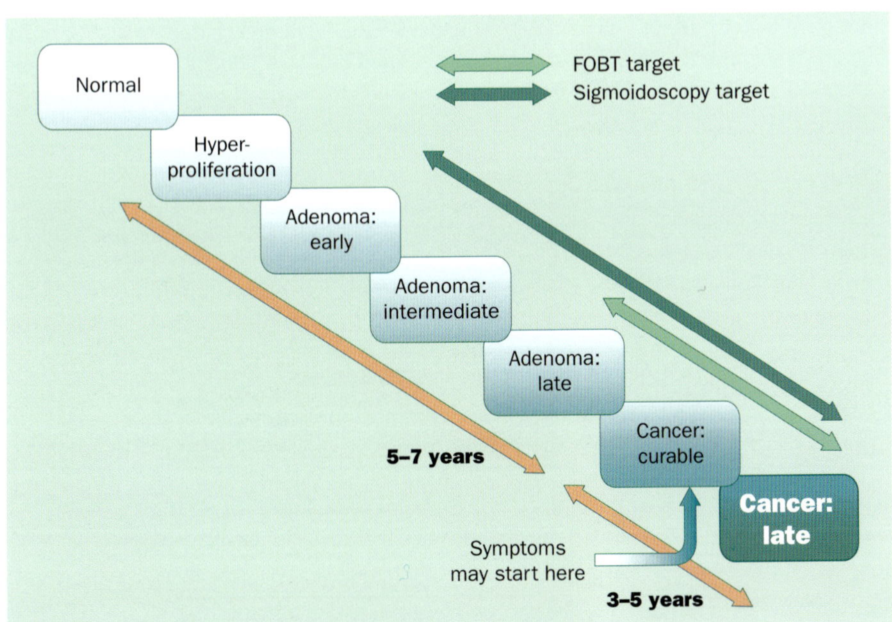

Figure 8.1 *The stages of colorectal tumorigenesis, their duration, their relationship to symptom onset, and their likelihood of detection by clinical screening methods. Adenoma: early, intermediate, late, refers to size, amount of villous elements, and degree of dysplasia.*

whole, especially where healthcare costs are shared across the community as in Canada, Australia, Scandinavia, the UK, and so on, this chapter will address screening from the population and personal perspectives.

The screening program

Screening can be defined as an ongoing process directed at asymptomatic individuals, which has the goal of reducing mortality from colorectal cancer.

Where the *general population* is the starting point, the process must:

(a) be able to identify those in whom screening is not appropriate;

(b) be able to identify those who need individualized surveillance and/or genetic testing;

(c) have its potential value and adverse effects explained to participants in an informed manner;

(d) have its outcomes continually monitored;

(e) be able to be resourced and afforded by those who manage the healthcare system;

(f) be attractive to those lacking interest or motivation.

Where the *individual* is the starting point, the same principles apply, except that the last point is much less of an issue. Furthermore, the strategy is not so much to achieve participation with any test (any test being better than none at all), but rather to ensure that the best test is undertaken.

Screening is a stepwise process (Table 8.1). At each step, a judgement is based on likelihood of outcomes, and should be able to be justified on the basis of evidence. Therefore, we shall analyze each step from operational and outcome perspectives.

Targeting individuals at risk

In a Western country, everyone over 50 years is considered to be at least at 'average risk', i.e. at a sufficiently high probability of having colorectal cancer to justify screening on the grounds of cost-effective outcome. Age 50 is the generally accepted starting point in the absence of any other risk factors, and is the recommendation of the American Cancer Society and most other international authorities.[5] The prevalence of colorectal cancer in the state of Victoria, Australia in a

Table 8.1 *The screening process*

- Target those at risk for colorectal cancer
- Invite participation in screening program
- Ensure that special circumstances such as symptoms or family history are identified early in the process
- Perform the screening test, which is safe, effective, acceptable, and affordable
- Use the result to identify those who should undertake the diagnostic process
- Ensure compliance with the appropriate diagnostic follow-up
- Ensure adequate subsequent treatment
- Offer rescreening at appropriate intervals
- Monitor the outcomes of the program

population of subjects aged 25–50 is 0.016%, compared with 0.2% for those in the next 25-year age span (50–75 years).

However, any unselected population will include subjects with symptoms who require diagnostic assessment and who are not suitable for population screening. There will also be those of above-average risk who require an individualized approach to surveillance (see Chapters 6 and 7). These will usually not be apparent when the target population is defined unless screening is being managed through a physician or medical interviewer. Table 8.2 summarizes these points.

Table 8.2 *Targeting those at risk*

- Those aged 50–75 years in a Western country are 12 times more likely to have colorectal cancer than those aged 25–50 years.
- Those older than 50 years require at least a basic screening program such as a fecal occult blood test
- Those at even higher risk are those with:
  - symptoms possibly due to colorectal cancer
  - at least one first-degree relative with colorectal neoplasia
  - a personal history of colorectal neoplasia or chronic inflammatory bowel disease
- Those at higher risk need to be identified, and given a personalized assessment and possibly more intensive surveillance

Participation in screening

The initial offer of screening can take various forms: mass population, screenee-initiated, and physician-initiated[6] (Table 8.3).

The latter two forms are sometimes referred to as 'case-finding', and are discussed later in this chapter. Mass population-based screening is by nature impersonal, but is likely to be systematic in its approach and more likely to improve outcomes at the population level.

When screening is offered, whether from a central co-ordinating facility in a population program or in the context of case-finding, it should:

(a) optimize access, for example by including dia-grammatic instructions and relevant language;

(b) simplify and maximize participation, for example by providing the stool-sampling device and any dietary instructions as part of the offer (see also the section below on acceptability of screening tests);

(c) explain the potential benefit of participation – i.e. the reduction in mortality from bowel cancer in the participants;

(d) identify the outcomes and subsequent action required – i.e. a positive test requires diagnostic follow-up while a negative test has limitations;

(e) explain the risks, namely missed cancers or com-plications of colonoscopy; it is important to indi-cate that the screening test is a selection process for colonoscopy that directs colonoscopy to those more likely to have cancer – it might not pick up everyone!

(f) encourage ongoing, future participation;

(g) obtain informed consent.[7]

The goal of the offer is to get the highest possible participation rate, since curable lesions (asymptomatic cancers and adenomas) will only be found in those who undertake testing.

Table 8.3 *Ways to offer screening*

- Mass (population-based) screening. Mass screening can be systematic and comprehensive, but is impersonal

- Individualized screening (case-finding):
  – screenee-initiated screening, or
  – physician-initiated screening
  Individualized screening is ad hoc, but ensures appropriate attention to personal situation

Organizing a screening program

Organization of a screening program can be at vari-ous levels: by a government health authority, by pre-ventive health personnel within a health maintenance organization (HMO) (see Table 10.8 in Chapter 10), or by the practitioner.

The first approach is illustrated by the model of national mammography screening programs that are being implemented in Western European and Scandi-navian countries, among others. There are few exam-ples of large-scale colorectal cancer screening programs of this type that have been, or are being performed (see Chapters 1 and 10). If such an orga-nizational framework were in place for breast cancer screening, it might be cost-beneficial to utilize it also for a similar national colorectal cancer screening pro-gram. It is important not to provide a competing serv-ice that might be perceived by women as less relevant for them and give them the impression that breast and cervical cancer screening is their priority and the only necessary preventive examinations. An added benefit of enrolling the female partner, who is often responsible for family health practices, is that she can then persuade her partner to also partici-pate in such a preventive program. This has been one of the points emphasized in the recent US public health campaign for colorectal cancer screening.

Another possible model for organizing colorectal cancer screening is that of a large group practice, which may be multidisciplinary or a single subspe-cialty, usually gastroenterologists. They may be pro-viding medical services for a defined geographic area or subcontracting a medical insurance or servicing large places of work. Colorectal cancer screening added to the standard medical services provided may be offered as an incentive to join that medical service, or to obtain a service contract.

Lastly, in many medical systems, including those of countries having a high risk for colorectal cancer, the individual primary-care physician takes full responsi-bility for preventive medical practices in adults. This is also discussed in detail in Chapter 10.

Screening test options

The screening test is a key element of a screening pro-gram: those being offered the test must be prepared to take it, and doing so should increase the chance of detecting a curable lesion. The test must be sensitive (i.e. it should detect an adequate proportion of diseased individuals) and specific (i.e. it should not subject healthy persons to excessive anxiety or extra testing).

Screening methods that might be considered for use are summarized in Table 8.4, which also shows what each is capable of detecting.

Correct usage is vital to success. The biology of bleeding from neoplasia dictates both the correct usage of FOBTs and their efficacy. The anatomical distribution of colorectal neoplasias (cancer and adenoma) determines the usefulness of the sigmoidoscopic approach.

Symptoms and digital rectal examination

The classic clinical presentations of colorectal cancer are described in Chapter 1.

Performance of digital rectal examination in those over 50 years of age seems prudent as part of any physical examination and certainly as part of a work-up for rectal bleeding. It should be performed before inserting an endoscope and should include examination of the prostate. Inclusion of an FOBT test on a sample obtained by digital rectal examination is not advisable because of the higher false-positive rate caused by lack of dietary preparation. Nonetheless, performing FOBT by this method may be better than not doing it at all.[8] Despite its frequent use for screening in the USA, it has not been rigorously tested in large groups of asymptomatic subjects. Indeed, it provides

just a single sample when other studies clearly demonstrate that two or three samples are desirable.

Fecal occult blood tests (FOBTs)

The fact that microscopic bleeding may arise from curable cancers provides the basis for screening based on FOBTs. However, the biology of bleeding is complex, and for FOBT-screening to be effective, these tests must be used properly in a way that maximizes their ability to detect bleeding from neoplasia.

Technological issues with FOBTs

FOBTs available for screening are based on two principal technologies: chemical tests and immunochemical tests (I-FOBTs). The major features of these tests[9] are outlined in Table 8.5. Key issues for their usage are outlined in Table 8.6. The main brands commercially available are listed in Table 8.7, but it must be emphasized that the levels of evidence supporting use of an individual brand vary greatly.[10]

The *chemical tests* (e.g. Hemoccult II) use guaiac to detect the peroxidase activity of heme (Tables 8.5 and 8.6).[11] Hence, they react to any peroxidases in feces (e.g. those in plant foods and heme in red meat) and are affected by certain chemicals (e.g. vitamin C). Because heme is relatively stable in the gut (although slow degradation occurs in the colon), these tests may detect bleeding from any site, including the stomach. The sample collection device for these tests requires the screenee to take a sample of feces, avoiding contamination by toilet bowl water, and smear the sample onto the device. In the laboratory, developing the card to read the result (qualitative) is simple (Figure 8.2), but might not always be completely accurate in practice without training. Hemoccult SENSA is deliberately made to be more readable (Figure 8.2) and more sensitive for peroxidase, but this may affect its specificity slightly.[12] It is now clear that if test development is delayed for 72 hours after sampling, the problem of plant peroxidase interference is minimized.[13] So dietary restrictions for guaiac tests can be simplified to exclude red meat and very high-peroxidase foods such as horseradish.

Before the availability of Hemoccult SENSA, rehydration of Hemoccult was introduced to improve sensitivity, but this has an adverse effect on specificity, by activation of plant peroxidases, and is no longer recommended.[10,13]

I-FOBTs use antibodies specific for human globin (Tables 8.5 and 8.6).[11] They are not affected by diet. Because globin is rapidly degraded by digestive enzymes, these tests are highly selective for occult colorectal bleeding.

Table 8.4 Options for screening methods	
Method	**Impact**
Digital rectal examination	Reaches 25–30% of rectal cancers
FOBT – guaiac	Detects microscopic blood in feces from entire gastrointestinal tract (cancer better than adenoma)
FOBT – immunochemical	Detects microscopic blood in feces as hemoglobin only, from colon/rectum (cancer better than adenoma)
Flexible sigmoidoscopy	Accurate detection for cancer and adenoma within reach (55% of all)
Colonoscopy	Accurate detection for cancer and adenoma within reach (95% of all)

Table 8.5 *Main features of different types of fecal occult blood tests (FOBTs)*

Type of FOBT	Basis	Stool-sampling method	Endpoint
Chemical	Guaiac; detects peroxidase	Wooden spatula and fecal smear for most	● Blue blush of color on paper card
Immunochemical	Anti-hemoglobin antibody	Wooden spatula, probe, spoon, or brush	● Latex or red cell agglutination ● Solid-phase immunochromatography ● Enzyme-linked immunosorbent assay (ELISA)

Table 8.6 *Usage issues for different types of fecal occult blood tests (FOBTs)*

Type of FOBT	Diet restrictions	Drug interference	Site of bleeding detectable	Endpoint for test result
Chemical	Must avoid red meats; possibly avoid certain raw plant foods[a]	Vitamin C; possibly NSAIDs[b]	Rectum > colon > stomach (in decreasing order of sensitivity)	● Subjective and transient[c]
Immunochemical	None required	None required	Colon and rectum	● Agglutination tests[c] – can be difficult to read ● Immunochromatography – easy to read ● ELISA – machine-read

[a] Delaying development for 72 hours minimizes interference from plant foods and avoids the need for their restriction.
[b] Non-steroidal anti-inflammatory drugs; low-dose aspirin is not a problem, but therapeutic doses for rheumatic disorders may be so.
[c] The tests generally provide a qualitative result, but newer immunochromatographic tests may be quantifiable.

Table 8.7 *Examples of commercially available fecal occult blood tests (FOBTs)*

Guaiac tests

● Hemoccult II, Hemoccult, Hemoccult SENSA (Beckman Coulter, Inc., Primary Care Diagnostics)

● Colo-Rectal (Hoffmann LaRoche AG)

● Seracult Plus (Propper Manufacturing Co., Inc.)

● HemoFEC (Boehringer Mannheim GmbH)

● ColoScreen (Helena Laboratories)

Immunochemical tests

● Immudia HemSp (Fujirebio, Inc.)

● Hemolex (Orion Diagnostica)

● Mono-Haem (Silenus Laboratories)

● FlexSure OBT, HemeSelect (Beckman Coulter, Inc., Primary Care Diagnostics)

● !nform, !nsure OBT (Enterix Australia and Enterix United States, respectively)

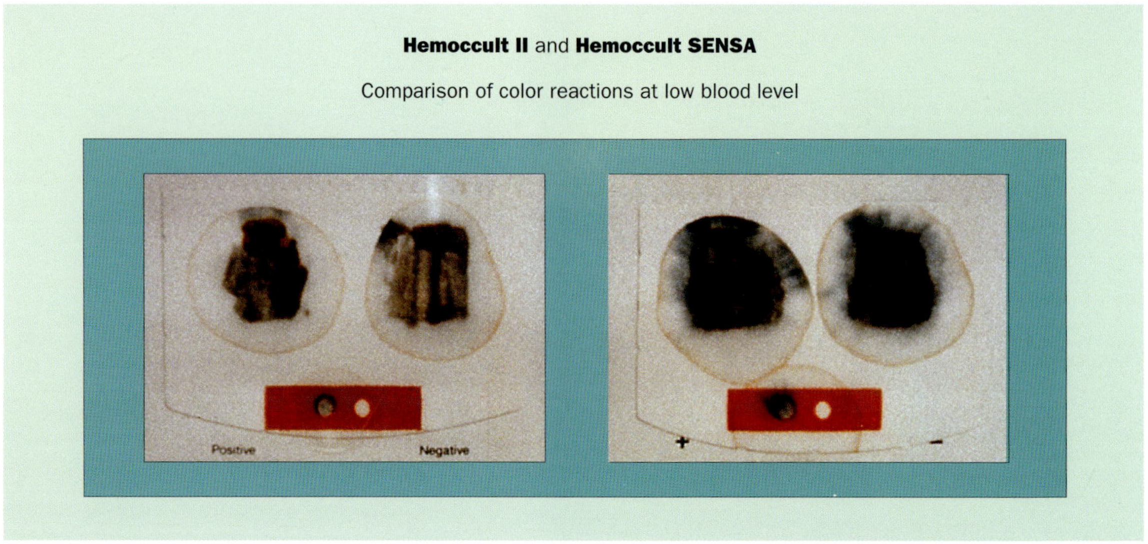

Figure 8.2 *Developed sample cards from Hemoccult II (left) and Hemoccult SENSA (Beckman Coulter, Inc.) (right). Note the more easily read Hemoccult SENSA. Blood levels in the stool were the same for each test.*

Depending on the version of FOBT and the manufacturer, improvements in fecal sampling have been made, although most still require very close contact with feces. For instance, Immudia HemSp uses a probe that is poked into the stool, while FlexSure OBT uses a stick-and-smear approach similar to Hemoccult. Readability is generally simple and reliable (Figure 8.3). While FlexSure OBT uses an immunochromatographic method similar to a urine pregnancy test, to give a qualitative result, Immudia HemSp requires laboratory development using a hemagglutination method. It is beyond the scope of this chapter to explore the technological details further, but laboratory development is preferred in many countries – especially for mass screening, when many tests must be done.[14]

A new generation of I-FOBTs has been released where development and reading is automated and the result is quantifiable. These include the MagStream HemSp development of Immudia HemSp and the !nform test. The advantage of measurement is that it returns full control of sensitivity and specificity to the end-user. In other words, those carrying out screening can select a value of fecal hemoglobin as the cutoff level that suits their population.

Bleeding from colorectal neoplasia

The nature of blood products excreted in feces varies according to the site of bleeding (Table 8.8).[11] I-FOBTs are advantageous, since they are more selective for large-bowel bleeding. While fecal blood loss is common in patients with colorectal neoplasia, it is not always outside the normal range of up to 1.5 ml/day,[15] and FOBTs will never completely discriminate between normal subjects and cancer-bearing patients (Figure 8.4).[16] Adenomas bleed less than cancers, and bleeding from small adenomas (<1 cm) is uncommonly outside the normal range.

Table 8.8 *Relationship between site of bleeding and type of fecal occult blood test, shown in relative terms and in approximate sensitivity (graded + to +++++) as milliliter of blood per day if lost in a single, discrete bleed[a]*

Type	Site		
	Gastric	**Cecal**	**Rectal**
Guaiac	+ (10–20 ml)	+++	++++ (0.5 ml)
Immunochemical	– (40–100 ml)	++/+++	+++++ (0.25 ml)

[a] Adapted from reference 11.

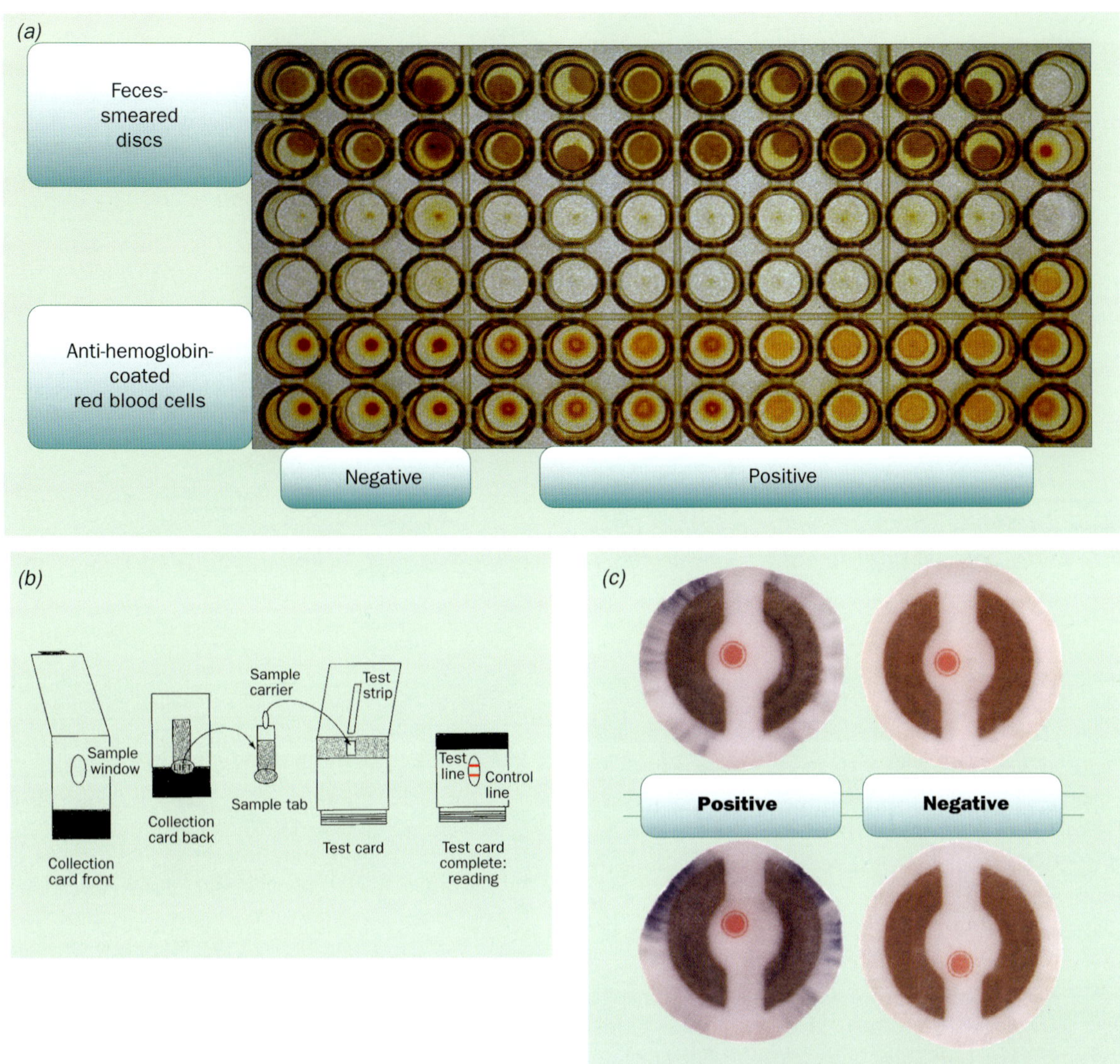

Figure 8.3 *Examples of developed immunochemical FOBTs. (a) Hemagglutination plate for the Immudia HemSp (and HemeSelect) test, showing positive and negative results. (b) Sample developed by the immunochromatographic method of the FlexSure OBT test. The Enterix OBT test gives a similar endpoint. (c) Latex agglutination results for Hemolex.*

Furthermore, the quantity of bleeding from cancers varies from day to day in patients with neoplasia, and so it is normally recommended that FOBTs be performed on multiple (usually three) separate stools.[11]

Thus, FOBTs primarily lead to detection of cancer, although they do facilitate detection of some larger adenomas.

Correct usage of FOBT

When subjects use an FOBT, it is important that they follow the manufacturer's instructions carefully. These usually describe how to achieve control of sample size and stability of sample for hemoglobin detection, and do not recommend obtaining the sample by digital examination. It is useful to provide a collecting device that facilitates stool sampling and avoids contact with toilet water and/or chemical cleaners. The stool-collecting device should be disposable in the toilet. Stool sampling should be performed by the screenee using the manufacturer's sampling device, with the sample being returned to the doctor or laboratory for development. Dietary restrictions (avoidance of red meat) should be followed if a guaiac

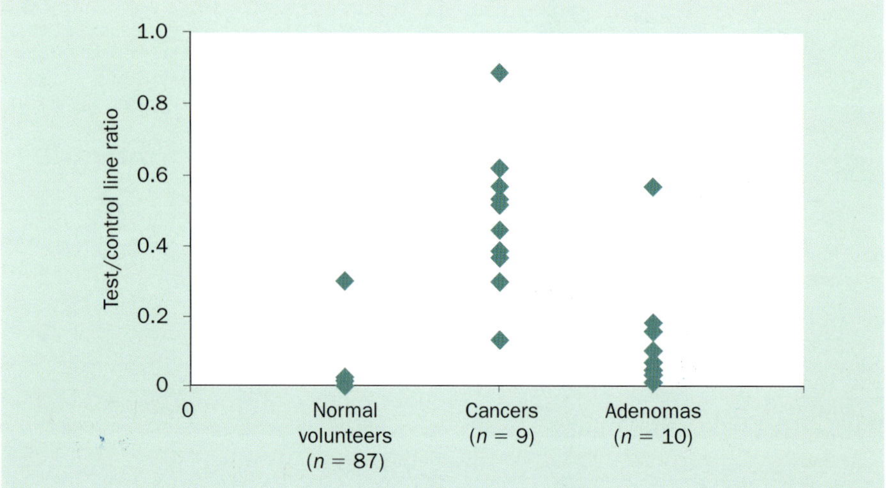

Figure 8.4 *Different levels of fecal hemoglobin as measured by a quantifiable immunochromatographic method (Insure OBT). Note the small overlap between normals and cancer patients, and the intermediate levels in those with adenomas.*[11]

test is used, and stools should be sampled from multiple points at the surface of each stool. These points are summarized in Table 8.9.

Summary

1. Two different types of FOBT are readily available; their requirements are different in practice.
2. Dietary factors and drugs may interfere with guaiac tests. The more sensitive guaiac tests are especially at risk of dietary false-positive results.
3. The type and quantity of blood derivatives in feces vary with the site of occult bleeding, and immuno-chemical tests are 'colorectal-selective'.
4. FOBTs will not completely discriminate between those with and without neoplasia.
5. The manufacturer's recommendations for sampling of stools should be followed closely, and samples should be sent to the office/laboratory in the sampling device and not as whole stools.
6. Contamination of feces by toilet bowl water before sampling should be avoided.
7. Multiple samples should be taken from the surface of the stool.
8. Multiple stools (at least two and preferably three) should be sampled.

Practical points when using an FOBT

The guaiac-impregnated test card is the most commonly used FOBT, outside of Japan. These are relatively inexpensive and there are various manufacturers (Table 8.7 of Chapter 8). Published quality control of sensitivity for known levels of fecal occult blood and the results of their use in clinical trials are the only objective means to decide which manufacturer's product to use.[10]

Preparing the FOBT card seems easy, but there are points to note that will help obtain maximum compliance for their use and quality performance. The first is to overcome the psychological barrier to manipulating feces. The use of an explanatory video film and/or personal explanation by a nurse–practitioner or medical interviewer can help overcome this initial barrier. English-language general educational materials on colorectal cancer screening are obtainable from Beckman Coulter Primary Care Diagnostics, Palo Alto, California (askpcd@beckman.com). They have also prepared an instruction video in major languages.

In order to facilitate compliance for screening and annual repeated FOBTs, the dietary and medication limitations should be minimized. These have been described in this chapter. Similarly, the collection of fecal samples should be as easy and as efficient as possible. This is best done by using a paper

Table 8.9 *Important points for correct usage of fecal occult blood tests (FOBTs)*

- Sampling of stools onto the sampling device should be performed by the screenee using the manufacturer's sampling device and following the manufacturer's instructions

- The manufacturer's instructions should also be used for storing and transporting samples

- Screenees should avoid straining at stool

- Menstruation, and sampling after participation in endurance sports, may give a positive result

- Dietary restrictions should be followed if a guaiac test is used, and should be commenced three days prior to taking the first sample; avoid taking vitamin C with guaiac tests

- Do not cease low-dose aspirin prescribed for cardiovascular disorders, but it is prudent to avoid larger doses of anti-inflammatory drugs (guaiac tests only)

- Stools should be sampled from multiple points at the surface of each stool

- Avoid contact of stools with toilet bowl water unless this is allowed by the sampling procedure

- Return the samples as quickly as possible for development

collecting device that can be attached to the toilet seat or toilet bowel (Figure 8.5). This allows for easier sampling, avoids contact with toilet water (and chemicals), and allows for disposal of the stools and collecting paper in the toilet.

Cards must be clearly identified with the screenee's name, etc., and the date of preparation (Figure 8.6). The thinly smeared cards should be left open for a few minutes until air-dried. This minimizes bacterial degradation of fecal hemoglobin and its products. For the same reason, completed cards should be kept in a cool place until returned for development. Special return mailing envelopes are available, but, even so, exposure to high ambient temperatures in an outdoor mailbox should be avoided.

These instructions are also applicable to immunochemical FOBTs that use a card similar to the guaiac test.

Practical points on developing the guaiac FOBT

The guaiac FOBT is frequently developed and interpreted by various non-laboratory-trained personnel. This is an error, since there are potential sources of mistakes that can lead to under- or over-reading of the test result. The clinical significance of a false-positive or false-negative test has been described in Chapter 1 and elsewhere in this chapter. Video films, in major languages, on developing and interpreting the guaiac test are also obtainable from Beckman Coulter. Points to note are as follows: develop the FOBT card no

sooner than 3 days after preparing the last test so as to allow degradation of vegetable peroxidases, but no later than 14 days after the first test preparation so as to prevent dehydration and loss of sensitivity. Expiry dates of developing agents need to be checked. The test card should have an internal control to demonstrate that the developing agents and the card itself are performing as expected. After applying the developing agent, a timer should be used and the card carefully observed for any transient positive (blue) coloration around the edges, or spreading out from the smeared 'window' (Figure 8.2).

It must be remembered that the final reading is subjective – namely the identification of a blue color. There are several sources of potential error. If the FOBT manufacturer has not maintained quality control of the background paper, it may be off-white and give a bluish tinge when wet with the developing agent. Bile staining will give a greenish color, and iron or bismuth a black color, to the smeared stools. Examples of developed FOBTs are shown in Figure 8.7, and these illustrate the range of colors that represent positive or negative tests for fecal occult blood when using the guaiac reagent.

For all the above reasons, in order to minimize subjective errors, it is best to centralize the development of FOBTs and have it done by experienced technicians. This also allows for quality control, which should be done once or twice a year by providing smeared cards that have had known amounts of blood added to normal feces. This also allows for the evaluation of the reading threshold of the technicians.[17]

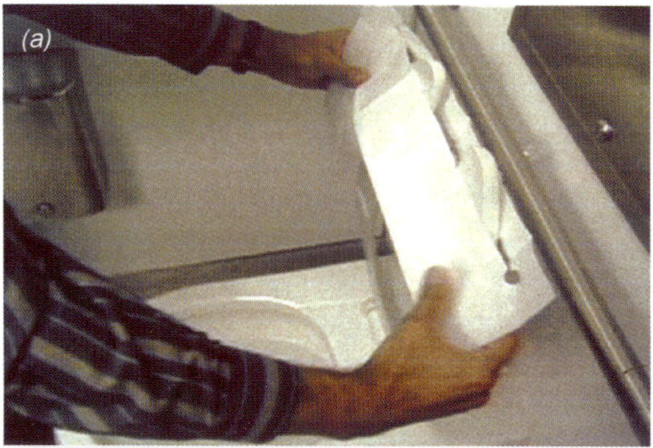

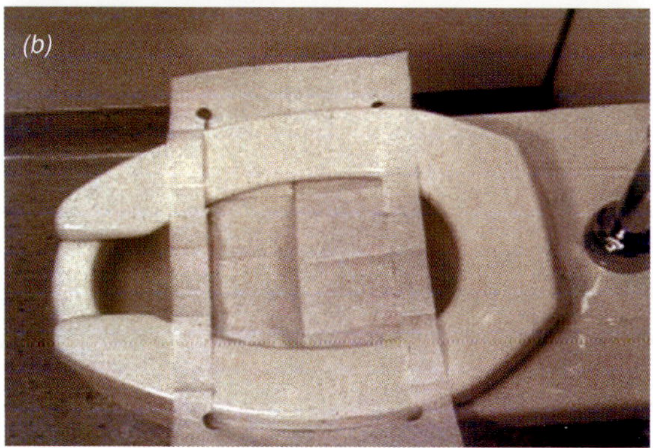

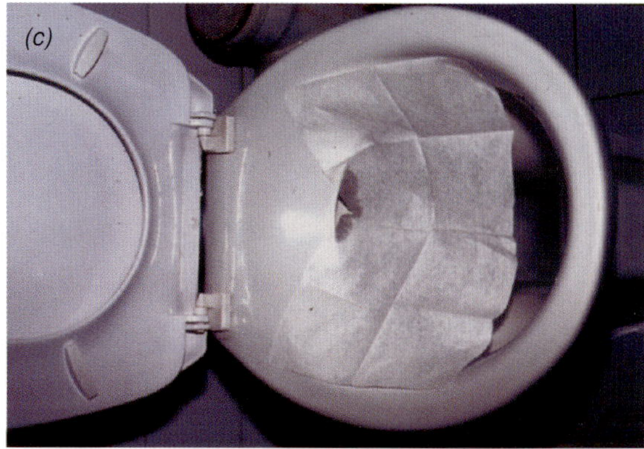

Figure 8.5 *(a) Applying the slip-on paper stool-collecting device to the toilet seat. (b) The stool-collecting device in place. (c) A different collecting device having adhesive corners that are attached to the sides of the toilet.*

Radiology

The use of a barium enema every 3–5 years as the screening tool has been considered to be a cost-effective strategy. Clearly, the quality of the examination and experience of the person interpreting the films is of great importance. The Council of the American College of Radiology has recommended a practice standard that allows detection of 90% of cancers and 80% of polyps larger than 1 cm.[18] This can best be achieved by quality, air-contrast studies.[19]

The sensitivity of barium enema will be better than that of FOBTs, but at greater initial financial cost, inconvenience, and complication rate (albeit very low). Radiology is relatively insensitive for identifying small polyps – a characteristic that might well be an advantage.[18] A recent comparison of colonoscopy and double-contrast barium enema for surveillance after polypectomy showed the former to be the more effective method.[20] In addition, there is little information available on the use of radiology as a mass-screening tool, and so compliance and willingness to return for repeated examinations are uncertain. Because there has not been a formal trial in population screening, its use cannot be recommended. As the methodology of virtual colonoscopy improves, this may become a feasible screening tool. For computed tomography (CT)-based virtual colonoscopy, bowel preparation is still required.

Sigmoidoscopy and colonoscopy

There are significant differences between using a test for diagnostic purposes and for screening purposes – a distinction that is often overlooked. A diagnostic test is applied to an individual, often with symptoms, where the likelihood of disease is relatively high and side-effects are easily balanced against the benefit. A screening test is applied to a

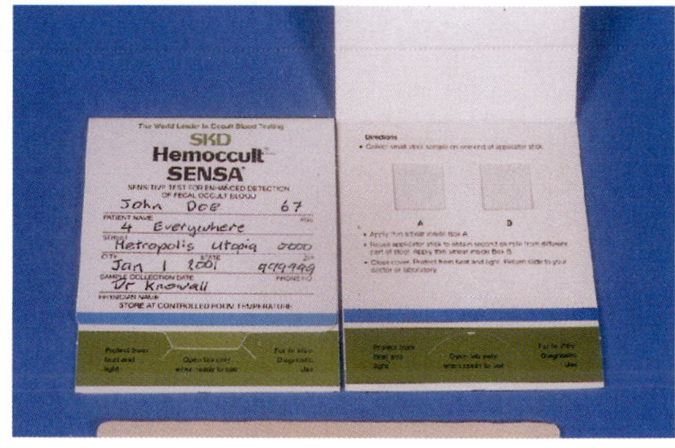

Figure 8.6 *The front of each FOBT card must be filled in with identification data and date. This flap is then opened and stools thinly applied to each of the two 'windows' using the wooden spatula provided. Other FOBTs use similar cards.*

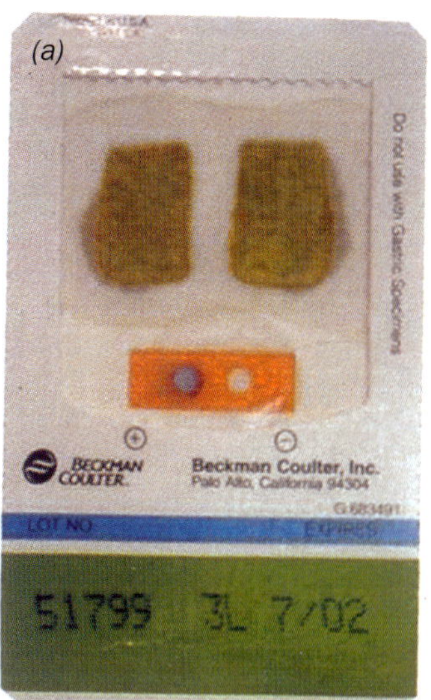

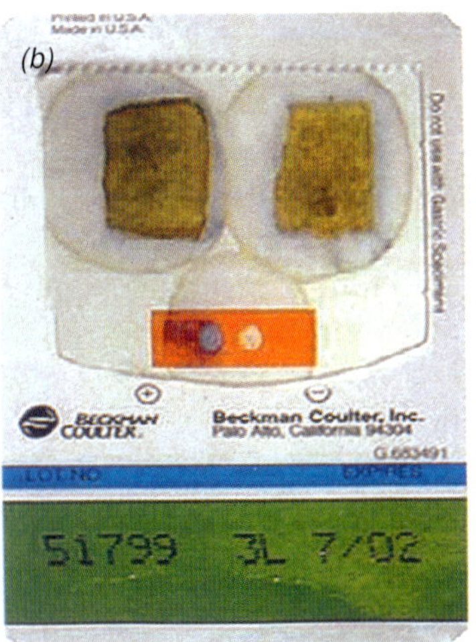

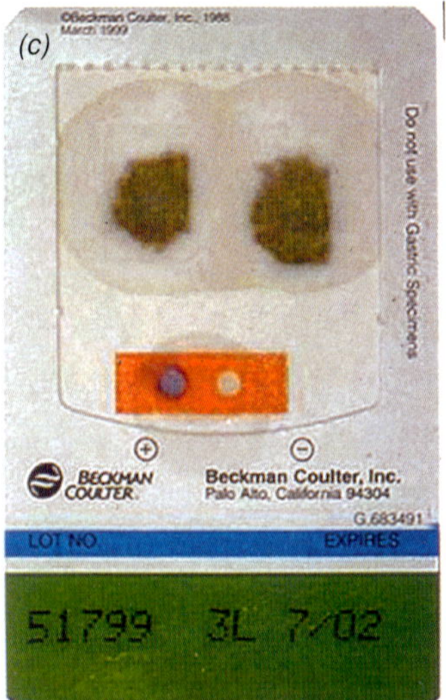

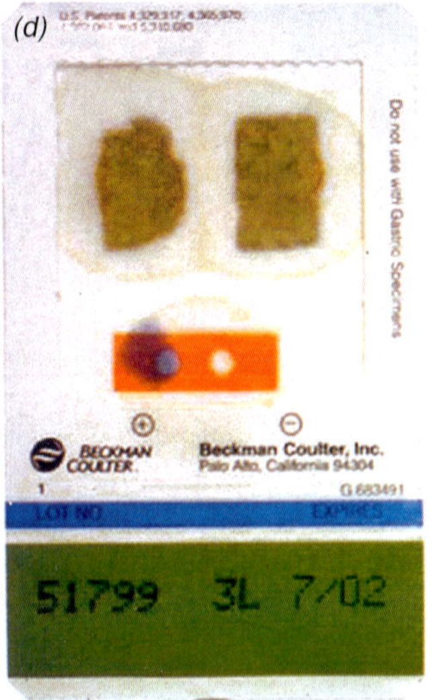

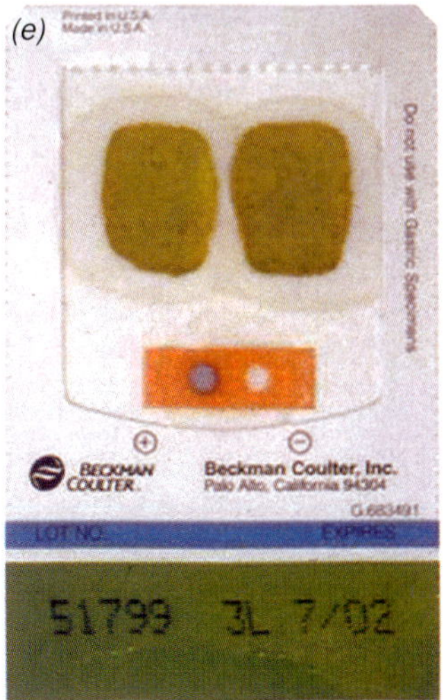

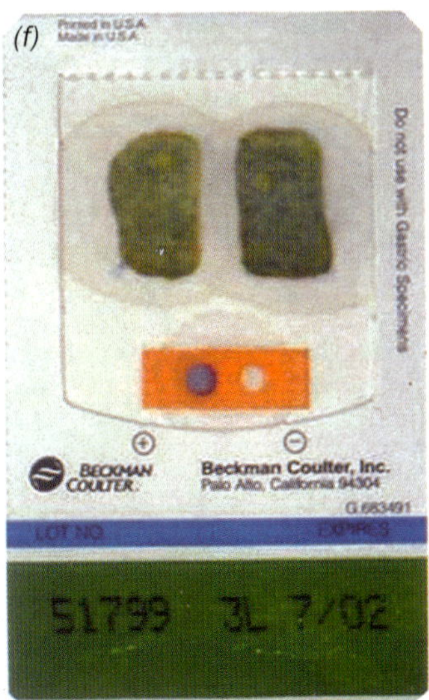

Figure 8.7 (a) Developed guaiac FOBT negative for occult blood. Note the blue color of the 'performance' monitor on the lower left and the lack of color on the lower right after applying the developing reagent. This indicates the correct performance of the test card and reagents. There is no blue color around the two smeared windows. (b) There is a strong blue color that has leached out around the smeared windows, indicating a positive test. (c, d) There is a weak bluish tinge around the smeared windows, still indicating a positive test. (e) Note the greenish tinge of the smeared 'windows' after applying the developing reagent. This is due to bile staining, and as there is no blue color, it is a negative test for blood. (f) After applying the developing reagent, there is both a green tinge due to bile and a surrounding bluish tinge indicating a positive test for blood.

well individual with low likelihood of disease where any level of complication could make it unacceptable. This distinction becomes critically important when considering endoscopic screening. On the other hand, endoscopic methods clearly improve the chance of detecting adenomas.

Rigid proctosigmoidoscopy

Rigid proctosigmoidoscopic examination is anatomically limited by distal rectosigmoid angulations, and often will not negotiate the rectosigmoid junction. In practice, it detects about 25–30% of colorectal cancers,[21] although a rate of 45% is theoretically possible based on recent UK data on distribution of cancers in the large bowel, if the rectosigmoid junction were always visualized.[22] It is rarely used as the sole screening tool, and is much less comfortable than flexible sigmoidoscopy.

No special facilities are required, although training in technique and lesion recognition is essential. Because of the diagnostic limitations and discomfort associated with this examination, it is not used as a screening test.

Flexible sigmoidoscopy

Flexible sigmoidoscopy (video or fiber-optic) achieves more comprehensive views of the rectum and sigmoid colon than the rigid proctosigmoidoscope. While 30 cm and 60 cm instruments are available, the longer is the most commonly used. Its field of view is greater, with its size and flexibility allowing more comfortable insertion and manipulation around the rectosigmoid junction and sigmoid colon than the rigid sigmoidoscope. Significantly more neoplastic lesions are identified than with rigid sigmoidoscopy, and (with the 60 cm instrument) one-half to two-thirds of neoplasms are within its reach in practice. This examination can be conducted without sedation and with enema preparation only, but the facilities required for instrument maintenance and disinfection are the same as those for colonoscopy. Instruments with a removable sheath have been developed that do not need disinfection. Information on one such product can be found at www.endosheath.com.

A detailed comparison of the usage and efficacy of rigid and flexible sigmoidoscopy has been reported by the American Medical Association.[23] Appropriate training and facilities are necessary, and nurses can be trained to perform flexible sigmoidoscopy. The technique has been described in detail.[24] A DVD has been prepared describing all aspects of the procedure (contact www.zephyrmedical.com for details) To help training in its performance, a simulator model has been developed to obtain initial experience before supervised and independent examinations. In order to promote its quality performance, the American

gastroenterology societies set up the Institute of Clinical Evaluation to certify training and knowledge of flexible sigmoidoscopy (www.icemed.org). Polypectomy should not be performed during sigmoidoscopic screening unless full bowel preparation has been performed or CO_2 insufflation is available.

Colonoscopy

Colonoscopy is the most accurate means of examining the colon. Combined with the ability to take biopsies and intervene therapeutically, it is the ideal diagnostic tool for follow-up after polypectomies[20]. However, the need for vigorous bowel preparation and sedation of subjects, the time lost from employment, the need for trained personnel, limited availability in many countries, and the relatively high cost make it of questionable cost-effectiveness as the primary screening tool for the average-risk subject. As with flexible sigmoidoscopy, appropriate training is essential, special facilities are necessary, and training in sedation is essential. This method is being evaluated as an alternative to FOBT and flexible sigmoidoscopy screening, especially since it is a more precise test and can examine the proximal colon.[25,26] Because of its clinical advantage over other screening tests, it has been accepted by the US Medicare Program as a screening test, available every 10 years, to the average-risk population, while the Italian Public Health Service allows it to be performed every 5 years (see Chapter 1).

Summary

1. The proportions of colorectal cancers reached by rigid or flexible sigmoidoscopy or colonoscopy are limited by their reach into the colon.
2. While preparation for colonoscopy is complex, only an enema is required for flexible sigmoidoscopy. Inconvenience ranks similarly.
3. The facilities required for the flexible endoscopic procedures are substantial.
4. Training is necessary for all procedures, but is most complex for colonoscopy.

Organizing screening sigmoidoscopy sessions

This can be efficiently organized by utilizing existing endoscopy services outside clinical hours, or by devoting them for this purpose at specific times. The advantages are to not mix the apprehensive healthy screenees with clinical patients whose test may be prolonged, sometimes complicated, and require use of recovery facilities. After clinical hours is frequently more convenient for the working screenee, while a dedicated morning session may be more convenient for those who work at home.

One of the main inhibitions to screening flexible sigmoidoscopy is the need for enema preparation. This can be done at home, but is most convenient if done en-suite, i.e. adjacent to the endoscopy rooms. This is especially important for persons traveling some distance before the test or coming after work. There is no need for dietary restrictions before examination, and the enemas can be self- or nurse-administered. The sigmoidoscopy examination should take less than 10 minutes, and the examinee does not need special clothing other than being draped to prevent soiling of clothes or embarrassment, nor is there need for recovery facilities.

An efficient screening session should last about 2 hours, and allow for the examination of about 10 persons. The team should consist of the medical interviewer–receptionist, cleaning–reprocessing technician, two nursing assistants (one assisting in preparing for screening and another helping during screening), and physician or nurse–practitioner screener (if the latter, then a physician should be easily available). Equipment should be on-hand for biopsy and photography of lesions. The latter is especially important when lesions are identified by nurse-practitioners. Video-endoscopy is advantageous for team observation and often useful for promoting screenee cooperation and understanding. The conditions should be calm and sympathetic so as to minimize the anxiety felt by the healthy screenee. These conditions will promote willingness for periodic recall examination and to persuade others to participate.

So as to minimize discomfort, it is important that an experienced endoscopist perform the test. The endoscopist can be a trained nurse–practitioner where this is allowed. They are not less efficient than a specialist physician–endoscopist, who is often unwilling to spend his or her expensive time on such preventive routine examinations.[27]

The most time-efficient method is to utilize several endoscopy rooms, so that the examiner can go quickly from one examination to another. This allows for at least four examinations to be performed in an hour. For efficiency, at least three endoscopic instruments should be available. This allows for cleaning and reprocessing of each endoscope, which takes at least 30 minutes.

The least efficient approach is to have sigmoidoscopy performed by the occasional endoscopist. There are endoscopy-training programs for primary-care physicians.[28] However, skills are easily lost if not used frequently. The other major disadvantages are the need to invest in endoscopy instruments, having available skilled nursing help, and the need for quality-controlled cleaning and reprocessing of expensive equipment. Using an endoscope that has a disposable external sheath can eliminate the need for cleaning, but is more expensive.

Follow-up of a positive screening test

A positive FOBT

Any positive FOBT sample warrants diagnostic evaluation, preferably by colonoscopy, but sigmoidoscopy plus double-contrast barium enema is an acceptable alternative. In practice, primary-care doctors have not adequately followed this direction, often attributing the cause to possible confounding factors such as hemorrhoids, lack of dietary compliance, participation in endurance sports, and menstruation. Even if a screenee should not have done the test (e.g. at the time of menstruation) or did not follow the diet, colonoscopic follow-up must be carried out. After a series of media promotions in Chicago, more than 54 000 FOBT kits were sent on request to asymptomatic persons. Of the 26% of the tests that were completed, more than one-third of those with positive tests failed to respond to repeated inquiries for follow-up, and another 20% had an incomplete diagnostic work-up after referral to a physician. Physician non-compliance can adversely affect the value of screening, and could be viewed as negligence.

A 'positive' sigmoidoscopy

The finding of an adenoma over 1 cm in diameter, a villous adenoma, or multiple adenomas at flexible sigmoidoscopy are the minimum requirements for colonoscopic follow-up.[29] Approximately 30% of cancers proximal to the splenic flexure have an index lesion situated more distally. Many argue on the potential sentinel status of a distal adenoma for proximal cancer or, on the basis of the adenoma–cancer sequence, that colonoscopic follow-up is required for all adenomas. As the follow-up colonoscopy rate could be as high as 25–35% with this recommendation, it will create a huge demand on resources. It also ignores the finding that not all distal adenomas, once removed, pose a risk now or in the future for cancer.[30] The current trial of flexible sigmoidoscopy in the UK should answer the question of what type of adenoma should trigger colonoscopic follow-up.

The principles of appropriate test follow-up are shown in Table 8.10.

Safety and adverse events

Safety is critically important when screening healthy people. Furthermore, the risks of screening are not just procedural but are also related to the anxiety that may be generated by increasing awareness of disease, by the delays between confirmation of potentially adverse findings, and by the relatively unseen adverse effects of missed cancers. Whichever screening tool is used, the mere process of public education and raised awareness of the possibility of disease in people who feel well has some consequences.[31]

Safety of FOBTs

FOBTs in themselves are quite safe apart from the small issue of hygiene. The consequences of testing create risks though. Following a positive test, there is a delay before colonoscopic follow-up that generates anxiety. If no neoplasia is found – a 'false-positive' test – then the anxiety may be viewed as having been unnecessary. But given that a clear colonoscopy indicates a very low risk for the next 5–10 years and probable lack of need for any screening during that time, it can be put in a positive light.

Following a negative test, a cancer may have been missed. This is inherent in the screening process. When screening is offered, it is important to indicate that the screening test is a selection process for colonoscopy that directs colonoscopy to those more likely to have cancer – it might not lead to the detection of all cancers!

Safety of radiology

The complication rate of barium enema is very low, although when perforation does occur, the mortality due to barium peritonitis is high. There is an issue of increasing exposure to radiation if this method is to be used repeatedly. As with FOBTs, any positive result must be followed up by colonoscopy to confirm the diagnosis of cancer by biopsy or to remove and evaluate the polyp. Hence the same principles of anxiety in anticipation and missed lesions apply as for FOBTs.

Safety of endoscopy

Screening flexible sigmoidoscopy appears to be particularly safe, since endoscopic biopsy is safe.[32] Sedation is not required for this procedure. Polypectomy should not be done unless CO_2 insufflation is available, and so the complications of bleeding and perforation are unlikely.

Widespread use of colonoscopy by non-expert operators could result in an increased complication rate and an increased rate of incomplete examinations. Careful quality control will be needed. The complication rate of screening colonoscopies is low: of 12 246 colonoscopies there were 4 perforations and 11 episodes of serious bleeding, i.e. a rate of major complications of about 1 in 800.[33]

Additional sources of anxiety created by colonoscopy are due to the delay between polypectomy and confirmation of histology and to the finding of an adenoma indicating increased risk and hence the need for ongoing colonoscopic surveillance. Its importance has never been clarified from the perspective of the participant.

Acceptability of screening tests

Acceptability of a test is critical to the success of screening. If a targeted person will not do it (i.e participate or comply with the offer), then, no matter how good the test, it will not be effective, since lack of participation clearly influences the ability of that test to detect neoplasia. Participation rates do differ between screening tools, and have to be considered in the context of a population-screening program. Observed rates for the screening tools are shown in Table 8.11.

Table 8.10 *Principles for follow-up of positive tests – 'positive' here refers to the result of a fecal occult blood test or the finding of an adenoma at sigmoidoscopy*

- Subjects should understand the action required for each test result when offered screening:
  - Negative result: come back again for rescreening at the correct interval; report any symptoms in the interim
  - Positive result: total colorectal evaluation is required
- The doctors involved must understand and implement these actions. Resources for follow-up must be available

Table 8.11 *Observed participation rates for various methods of screening when applied to average-risk subjects or populations*

Screening method	Participation rates
Digital rectal examination	Unknown
Fecal occult blood test	
● Done by physician	Unknown
● Provided as mass screening	50–70%[33–36] normally about 60%
Flexible sigmoidoscopy	
● Done by physician	Unknown
● Provided as mass screening	20–70%, normally 20–40%[37,38]
Colonoscopy	
● Done by physician	Unknown
● Provided as mass screening	6%,[39] 69%[26]

Acceptance of FOBT

Occult blood testing demands handling of feces in some way. Aversion to inspecting sampling, and handling feces is common in many societies. Available sampling methods are summarized in Table 8.12, and include making a smear of feces onto a test card with a stick, scooping or inserting a probe into feces and placing it into a screw-capped jar, throw-in-the-bowl methods, and wiping the anus with a sampling pad. This last method has poor clinical specificity. Throw-in-the-bowl, self-reporting tests are of concern with regard to the accuracy of interpretation of color in the bowl, the onus on follow-up action for a positive results remaining totally with the screenee, and reported lower sensitivities than Hemoccult for a number of these tests. Population-screening studies have shown that, despite the need for some dietary restriction, participation in guaiac-based FOBT screening is 55–70%.[33–36] The collection of portions of stool in jars without protease-enzyme inhibitors is to be discouraged, since it can lead to false-negative results because of enzymatic degradation of hemoglobin.[11]

Acceptance of sigmoidoscopy and colonoscopy

With screening by flexible sigmoidoscopy, participation rates in true mass-population studies vary from 20%–70%,[37,38] with 30–40% seeming to be a reasonable goal at present in a typical Western population. A rate of 70% has been achieved in population studies in Norway (Dr G Hoff, personal communication), which suggests that with education and encouragement, better participation rates are possible. Flexible sigmoidoscopy is more invasive and inconvenient than FOBT, and hence one suspects that compliance with the former will never be as good for mass screening when a physician or counsellor is not included, but this remains to be fully explored.

With colonoscopy, there has been no population screening study. In a study where screening colonoscopy was offered to physicians and dentists, participation was 6%.[39] In a more recent US study of screening colonoscopy offered to veterans (mainly men) at average and increased risk (family history of colorectal neoplasia), the acceptance was 69%.[26]

Table 8.12 *Available sampling methods for fecal occult blood tests, and their stability*

● Relatively stable methods
    Making a smear of feces onto a test card with a wooden spatula (e.g. Hemoccult SENSA)
    Dry-probe sampling methods (e.g. Immudia HemSp)

● Uncertain methods
    Scooping feces into a plastic jar
    Throw-in-the-bowl methods
    Wiping the anus with a sampling pad

● Innovative methods
    Brushing surface of stool immersed in toilet bowl

Effectiveness of screening tests

Parameters of effectiveness

Various traditional parameters are used to describe the performance of screening tests, and are similar to those used for diagnostic tests.[40] They include sensitivity, specificity, predictive values, and likelihood ratios. While all are relatively theoretical, each relates to a useful outcome or concept.

With population screening, a series of more practical outcomes needs emphasis:

- To influence mortality, we must be able to detect curable cancers and/or adenomas. Hence the overall detection rate or 'yield' of cancers in a screening program is vital.
- To be cost-effective and practical at a resource level, the rate of colonoscopic follow-up is vital. Hence the test positivity rate is important.

Ultimately, it is important that the screening tests lead to the performance of a sufficient number of colonoscopies to detect enough curable cancers and removable adenomas so as to reduce mortality at the population level.

Reduced mortality in FOBT screening

The value of FOBT-based screening is supported by the highest quality of evidence, namely three randomized controlled trials of screening, which have allowed for participation rates, have included systematic, unbiased ascertainment of participants, and have used mortality as the endpoint.[33–36] Results are summarized in Table 1.5 in Chapter 1. On an intention-to-screen basis, biennial screening with a guaiac-based FOBT (Hemoccult unrehy-

drated) reduces mortality by 15–20%, while annual screening (rehydrated Hemoccult) reduces mortality by 35–40%.[33,36]

On a participatory basis (i.e. based on those who actually perform the screening test), mortality is reduced by 40%.[34] FOBT-based screening acts primarily by facilitating colonoscopic detection of cancers at earlier stages. Yet, 18 years after commencing screening with annual rehydrated Hemoccult, not only does community mortality fall but so does incidence. Clearly, some adenomas are detected and removed as a result of detection of fecal occult blood, and this is not due to serendipitous detection at colonoscopy.[36]

These studies clearly demonstrate the benefit of FOBTs as a means of reducing mortality at the population and individual level. Not only do they do it by detecting early-stage cancer, but, with the more sensitive tests, they lead to adenoma detection and removal, which results in a reduction in cancer incidence as well.[36]

Cancer yield: a product of participation, sensitivity, and follow-up

Mortality reduction depends on the cancer yield of the screening program; it is the product of participation rate, sensitivity of the test, and compliance with follow-up. As such, sensitivity and participation rate are surrogate markers for impact on mortality. The interactive effect of participation and sensitivity is demonstrated in Table 8.13. It can be seen that even colonoscopy with its excellent sensitivity can be quite ineffective at the population level when participation is low.

Sensitivity of FOBTs

Despite the lower sensitivity of FOBTs, varying from 50%–90% depending on the type and frequency of screening,[33–36] they come out well in this intention-to-screen

Table 8.13 Impact of participation in the initial screening test and sensitivity of the test on yield of cancers in the program (rates given are representative of the literature)

Screening method	Sensitivity (%)	Participation rate (%)	Cancer yield in program (%)
Fecal occult blood testing	90	78	70
	55	60	33
Flexible sigmoidoscopy	75	60	45
	65	40	26
	55	20	11
Colonoscopy	95	6	6

analysis. The sensitivity of a once-off FOBT actually compounds with repeated testing. For instance, if a cancer remains at a curable stage for three years, then there are three opportunities to detect it by annual testing, and a 50% sensitivity for any once-only test compounds to 87.5%.

The sensitivity of Hemoccult can be increased with either hydration (which actually activates plant peroxidases, and is not to be recommended, since its disadvantages outweigh its advantages[13]) or with the enhanced reagents used for Hemoccult SENSA.[12] However, with both, the specificity is reduced by red meats and plant peroxidases, although the effect is not as great for Hemoccult SENSA and can be minimized.[13,17]

The sensitivity of immunochemical FOBTs (especially Immudia HemSp and HemeSelect) is better than that of Hemoccult, without unacceptable worsening of specificity.[41] As these tests do not require dietary restriction, participation rates are better, and so cancer yield will be substantially improved at the population level. Until now, their higher unit cost compared with Hemoccult has restricted their more widespread usage outside Japan.[10]

Choice of FOBT

At a population level, the ease of use of immunochemical tests gives them an advantage, but, at present, their cost creates difficulties. Table 8.14 lists the type of FOBT to be used in a particular population setting.[10]

Reduced mortality with sigmoidoscopic or colonoscopic screening

Recent case–control studies demonstrate an association between sigmoidoscopic examination of the rectum[21] or rectosigmoid[42] and a reduction in the chance of dying from colorectal cancer within reach. A case–control study from the Oakland Kaiser-Permanente program examined the use of screening rigid sigmoidoscopy,[21] and found that only 8.8% of the cancer patients had undergone screening sigmoidoscopy, compared with 24.2% of the controls – i.e. a risk reduction of 70% for *cancers within reach*. The data suggested that screening sigmoidoscopy may provide a risk reduction for as long as 10 years. Another case–control study found that a history of screening flexible sigmoidoscopy was present in 10% of those who died of colorectal cancer but in 30% of case controls – a reduction in the risk of death from colorectal cancer of 79%.[42] There have been no population-screening studies as yet, but they are in progress.

Because of the distribution of cancer in the large bowel, the sensitivity of sigmoidoscopy depends primarily on the depth of insertion. The skill of the operator, the adequacy of bowel preparation, and anatomy determine depth. Figure 8.8 shows the distribution of cancer in the colon based on data on new cancer diagnoses during 1988 in the UK.[22] It can be seen that if flexible sigmoidoscopy were to reliably include the splenic flexure, then approximately 73% of colorectal cancers would be detected directly. Experience with screening sigmoidoscopy has

Table 8.14 *Matching type of screening test to available facilities for evaluation*[a]

Where colonoscopic or sigmoidoscopic screening is not feasible or accessible

Colonoscopy resources for follow-up	Population compliance with diet for guaiac tests	Suggested FOBT
Unavailable		Do not screen
Limited	Generally good	High-specificity guaiac test (e.g. Hemoccult II)
Limited	Poor or uncertain	Immunochemical test
Readily available	Generally good	A sensitive guaiac test (e.g. Hemoccult SENSA)
Readily available	Poor or uncertain	Immunochemical test

Where sigmoidoscopic screening is feasible or accessible but colonoscopic screening is not

- Consider use with or instead of fecal occult blood test
- Choose complementary fecal occult blood test according to above table

Where colonoscopic screening is feasible and accessible

- Consider instead use of fecal occult blood test and/or flexible sigmoidoscopy

[a]Adapted from reference 10.

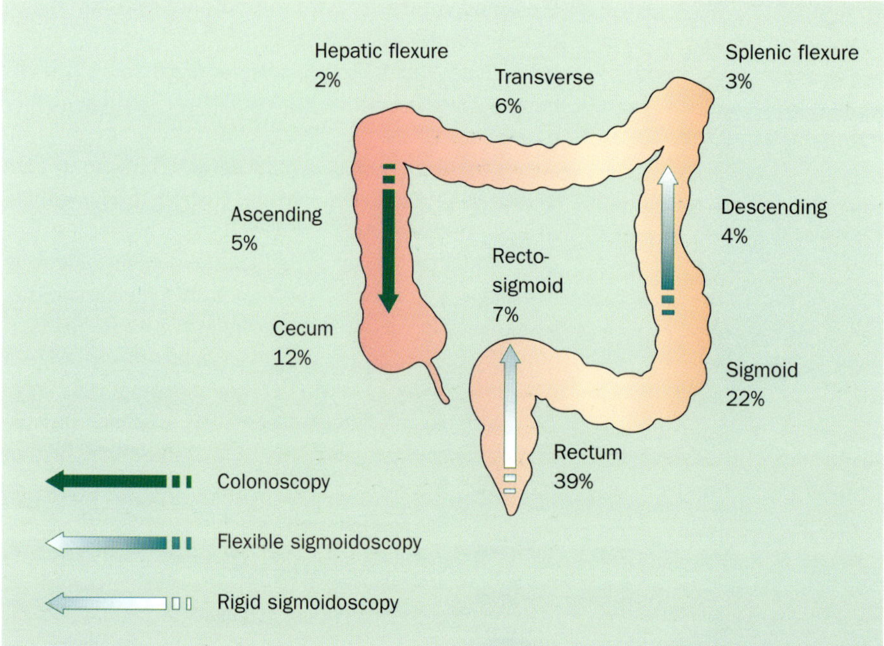

Figure 8.8 *Diagrammatic representation of the sensitivity of the various endoscopic methods according to reach around the colon[43] and percentage distribution of cancer.[22]*

been reviewed by Neugut and Pita.[43] In practice, the sensitivity of flexible sigmoidoscopy for cancer and large adenomas is in the range 33–60%.

At flexible sigmoidoscopy, 10–25% of screenees will have an index adenoma,[43] which means that the colonoscopic follow-up rate will be high. Given that approximately 30% of cancers proximal to the splenic flexure have an index lesion situated more distally,[44] one-third of cancers not seen at sigmoidoscopy seem likely to be picked up at subsequent colonoscopy, which would take the overall sensitivity of screening flexible sigmoidoscopy to 44–80%. This is similar to but not better than the sensitivity of guaiac FOBT!

With colonoscopy, it is theoretically possible to visualize the entire colon, and in expert hands this is possible in over 95% of occasions.[45]

Figure 8.8 summarizes the sensitivities of the various endoscopic methods according to reach around the colon. Note that the sensitivity of various types of FOBT in large population studies varies from 35% to 90% when they are used annually or biennially and depending on whether this is a one-time test or a repeated testing program over several years.

Combining FOBT and sigmoidoscopy

The combination of FOBT with flexible sigmoidoscopy has intuitive merit because they have complementary benefits – one being capable of detecting cancer at any level and the other adding more accurate adenoma and cancer detection within reach.[11] Adequate population trials have not been done to show the incremental benefit, and despite some calculations of cost-effectiveness suggesting it to be acceptable, the colonoscopic follow-up rate will be high.

Summary

1. The sensitivity of a screening method is critical to its impact on mortality, but must not be considered in isolation from the corresponding population participation rate.
2. Willingness to perform a test must be considered when predicting impact on mortality.
3. At present, participation with FOBT is better than demonstrated participation with sigmoidoscopic or colonoscopic screening.

Costs and cost-effectiveness

The initial costs of screening are largely due to the provision of FOBTs and the colonoscopies generated by positive tests (much the larger cost).[46] The test positivity rate (TPR) is thus a critical parameter. The TPR is the total of true positives (prevalence of disease times sensitivity) plus false positives (the inverse of specificity).

FOBT positivity rates

Immunochemical FOBT TPRs are unaffected by diet. Those for the best studied (Immudia HemSp and Heme-Select) are in the range 2–5%, a manageable rate for most Western populations.[41]

With guaiac-based FOBTs, additional problems arise. Confounding factors have been discussed in detail elsewhere, and are summarized in Tables 8.5 and 8.6. Plant peroxidases can give false-positive results, whereas vitamin C can cause false-negative results. Iron probably does not cause positive reactions. It is critical that red meat consumption be restricted for the more sensitive guaiac tests such as Hemoccult SENSA, and this is desirable for the less sensitive guaiac tests (e.g. Hemoccult), especially in populations where red meat consumption is high (e.g. USA, Canada, Australia, and New Zealand).

Positivity rates are reviewed in detail elsewhere.[10] For Hemoccult II in large studies, they have generally been in the range of 1–5%. Better sensitivities occurred with the higher TPRs. For rehydrated Hemoccult, the sensitivity can be 8–13%. For Hemoccult SENSA, TPRs are intermediate between these values.

Conclusion

It is now apparent that a better balance of TPR and sensitivity is achievable with I-FOBTs but these are more expensive than guaiac tests ($10–25 compared with $6–10 for three fecal samples), and costs are not always recoverable in healthcare systems around the world.

Sigmoidoscopy positivity rates

Depending on the age group and national dietary habits, 5–25% of screenees will have an index adenoma at flexible sigmoidoscopy, which means that the colonoscopic follow-up rate will be high for sigmoidoscopic screening. It should not be assumed that all polyps are adenomas. Not performing pathological examination on adenomas prior to scheduling colonoscopic follow-up of a polyp creates a major problem of specificity, and should be discouraged. About 50% of polypoid lesions will be non-neoplastic, i.e.

the observation of a polyp is 'false-positive' for neoplasia half the time. Given the evidence that subjects with a small distal tubular adenoma, once removed, are not at increased risk for cancer, surveillance colonoscopy may be ineffective in this group, and so small adenomas represent a problem of specificity in the context of cancer mortality reduction.[30] A randomized trial confirming the value of adenoma removal according to type, size, and number is now in progress.[47]

Cost-effectiveness

For colorectal cancer screening to be acceptable as formal public health policy, its cost-effectiveness must be of the same order as that of other cancer-screening programs that are already in place. A number of modeling studies in the USA, UK and Europe, and Australia have shown that the cost per life-year saved by FOBT screening is in the range $10 000–40 000, and is similar to that of breast cancer screening.[46,47]

Unfortunately, the costs of endoscopic screening will be considerable, owing to the cost of the initial screening test, the higher colonoscopic follow-up rate, and the competition for other healthcare resources. Calculations of cost-effectiveness of endoscopic screening provided so far,[48] while promising, are theoretical and suffer from the lack of real outcome data such as have been used to calculate cost-effectiveness for FOBT screening. Formal trials are clearly indicated.

Identifying those who will have the target lesion

The detection of blood is not intended to be the definitive diagnostic procedure, but rather to identify those more likely to have colorectal neoplasia at the present moment in time (see Table 8.15). This concept is embodied in the pre-test : post-test likelihood ratio, i.e. the chance of having colorectal cancer when one returns an abnormal test result.[11] It is simply the sensitivity of a test divided by its false-positive rate. It

Table 8.15 *Factors that influence an individual's likelihood for having colorectal cancer*

- Age: exponential rise beyond 45–50 years of age
- Personal history of adenoma or cancer: increases risk by a 3- to 7-fold increment
- Family history: increases risk by a 2- to 6-fold increment (even higher in the dominantly inherited syndromes)
- Fecal occult blood test: a positive result increases chance 11- to 45-fold relative to a negative test

provides a robust way of describing the effect of the test, because it is not affected by prevalence of cancer in the target population. Based on the sensitivity and specificity data using hydrated Hemoccult from the Minnesota controlled trial of screening (90.4% and 92.2%, respectively), the likelihood ratio is 12. Using an approximation of sensitivity (50%) and specificity (99%) from the Danish controlled trial of screening with standard Hemoccult, the likelihood ratio is 50. Such predictors of likelihood for cancer are obviously better than any other, including age and family history.

In other words, screening by FOBT leads to colonoscopy targeted at those more likely to have a neoplasm.

Endoscopic screening, where selection is based just on age, is random compared with FOBT-based screening, and more procedures will be done on people without neoplasia. With FOBT, the predictive value of a positive test for cancer is 5–10%.[33–36] Random colonoscopy in a population over 50 years would detect about 3 cancers per 1000. This is a predictive value of 0.3%, or one-tenth to one-twentieth that of FOBT.

When screening for colorectal cancer, the target lesions are curable cancers and removable adenomas – especially those cases with multiple adenomas, an adenoma larger than 1 cm, or an adenoma containing villous change. FOBTs largely target detection of curable cancer (Figure 8.1), although the Minnesota study shows some reduction in incidence due to adenoma removal. Visualization by endoscopy obviously improves adenoma detection, although how reliable it is remains to be seen, since some studies indicate that flat adenomas and 'de novo' cancers are more important than previously accepted.[49] How much value adenoma removal adds to the benefit of FOBT-based screening at the population level, where compliance will be different between the two modalities, remains to be demonstrated.

Rescreening

The complete screening program requires ongoing participation, preferably annually for FOBTs and every 5 years for sigmoidoscopy. It is critical that the screening process checks subjects for symptoms, personal history of colorectal neoplasia, or family history of colorectal neoplasia, and ascertains the presence of multisystem or serious disease where screening is irrelevant. The outcomes that might occur are thus the following:

1. Unwell – exclude from screening.
2. Symptomatic – send for diagnostic testing.
3. Personal history – provide colonoscopic surveillance at the correct interval.
4. Family history – profile actual risk and design a personalized surveillance program.
5. Flexible sigmoidoscopy negative – repeat in 5 years, with intervening annual FOBTs.
6. Flexible sigmoidoscopy shows neoplasia – for cancer, operate; for adenoma, perform colonoscopic polypectomy and plan ongoing surveillance at the correct interval.
7. Fecal occult blood test negative – repeat at 1-year (preferable) or 2-year intervals, advise need to report symptoms appearing in the interval.
8. Fecal occult blood test positive – full diagnostic evaluation of colon; in the absence of symptoms and iron deficiency, upper gastrointestinal endoscopy is not indicated if colonoscopy is negative.

Rescreening is important for all outcomes except the first. It is especially important for a negative FOBT or flexible sigmoidoscopy, since either may miss a cancer and repeated screening increases the chance of detecting this while still curable.

Individual choice and public responsibility in screening

For the individual seeking care (sometimes called case-finding) rather than being offered screening as part of a population mass-screening program, the key difference is motivation and willingness to undertake the test and ability of the healthcare system to resource the test that is agreed upon. For the population, doing something is better than nothing. For the individual, doing what is best is the issue, but cost and safety have to be considered.

Screenee-initiated screening and physician-initiated screening are the two mains forms of case-finding. Involvement of healthcare practitioners (e.g. primary-care physicians) has advantages in that there should be better motivation of the subject, symptomatic subjects are redirected from screening to appropriate diagnostic investigations, the screenee's risk status can be assessed prior to the choice of screening tool, and those at low risk because of age are excluded. Furthermore, the ongoing screening program can be tailored to the nature and degree of risk of the individual. The process is the same as in Table 8.1, but highly personalized and augmented by the encouragement from the physician involved.

Counselling about screening must include explanation of the following:

- There are three options in those over 50 years (FOBT and/or flexible sigmoidoscopy, or colonoscopy).
- There is proven value for the participant in repeated annual FOBT screening (mortality reduction of 40% or more for those who do it).
- FOBT screening acts as a selection process for those who benefit most from colonoscopy.
- Negative tests should not give false reassurance, and ongoing participation and early response to new symptoms are essential, since cancer can be missed.
- A positive test requires diagnostic follow-up.
- The risk of major complication from colonoscopy is about 1 in 800.
- Informed consent is based on provision of the above.

Relevant screening documentation and medical responsibility

It is essential that a medical interviewer or the physician obtain and document minimal medical information before initiating screening. This includes family history of neoplasia and past medical history of important gastrointestinal or other diseases or symptoms that could change screening methodology or even make screening irrelevant for that person. Before initiating screening, it must be made clear to the screenee that neither FOBT nor sigmoidoscopy, not even both screening tests together, can be absolute, and, even within a screening program (usually a 5-year cycle), they do not identify all colorectal neoplasia. So, screenees should be warned that if symptoms appear, they need to be investigated promptly. These points should appear on the informed-consent form.

Records should be computerized, and at the end of the session provide a report for the examinee and primary-care physician and allow for recall or follow-up to be arranged according to the established protocol. The importance of routine recall tests should be emphasized. In the case of a positive finding at flexible sigmoidoscopy or a positive FOBT, the scree-

nee must be notified personally, and this is recorded in the medical file. Failure to appear at a follow-up test should be recorded, including attempts to contact the patient personally.

When providing a final report, it is often beneficial to combine it with general preventive health recommendations. These relate to diet, tobacco smoking and alcohol consumption, weight control, mammographic screening, and routine gynecological examinations. This can be given by the examining physician, or in a busy practice by a nurse–practitioner or trained medical interviewer. The advice is usually well appreciated, and can be followed up by the primary-care physician (see Chapter 10).

National recommendations

National bodies throughout the world have varied in their willingness to concede that population-based screening for colorectal cancer is, as yet, justified.[3,10] For a health-care system, there are two key questions: Should it allow reimbursement for individual screening and/or should it implement an effective population policy?

Two countries have a population policy; Japan's is effective, but Germany's has limited acceptance, especially in men. The USA has now approved reimbursement, but does not have a national policy of implementation. Recently, in the USA, the Agency for Healthcare Policy and Research in association with five national medical societies, the American Cancer Society, and the US Preventive Services Task Force separately issued guidelines for colorectal cancer screening.[5] Other countries, such as Australia and the UK, are planning pilot studies to test the feasibility of implementation, while yet others, such as New Zealand, have rejected even pilot studies. Canada is reviewing its position. In Israel, FOBT screening is available upon request to every person after the age of 50 years. Endoscopic screening is available for all persons at increased risk because of family history or personal past history of premalignant disease.[3] In Italy, colonoscopy is now available as a screening test once in 5 years for the average-risk population (personal communication, Dr M Crespi, Rome).

Given that FOBT screening has been shown to be of proven efficacy by the highest level of evidence, and that sigmoidoscopic screening also has clear support, screening should at least be accessible to the individual, even if formal population programs are not funded.

Conclusions

The published data indicate that mortality from colorectal cancer can be reduced by annual FOBT programs (randomized controlled trials), which provide a 15–38% reduction on an intention-to-screen basis at the population level or at least a 40% reduction at the individual level when participation occurs. There is less strong evidence (case–control studies) for screening sigmoidoscopy, which provides a reduction that appears greater at the individual level but applies particularly to lesions within reach and perhaps relates to their better ability to detect adenomas. Nonetheless, sigmoidoscopy and colonoscopy add the benefit of improved adenoma detection; what remains unclear is how much added benefit there is and at what cost.

The American Cancer Society, the US National Cancer Institute, and several other groups around the world, including the National Cancer Control Initiative in Australia, recommend that screening for colorectal cancer begin at 50 years of age in average-risk persons. The US bodies recommend that it consist of annual FOBTs and/or flexible sigmoidoscopy every 5 years. Positive screening examinations should be followed by colonoscopy or, alternatively, double-contrast barium enema with sigmoidoscopy (preferably flexible). In practice, where there is face-to-face interaction between the doctor and the potential screenee, the options of FOBT with or without flexible sigmoidoscopy, flexible sigmoidoscopy alone, and even a colonoscopy should probably be discussed where these are accessible. However, the risks should also be carefully explained, and the imperative to do no harm must be carefully applied when screening the asymptomatic person.

References (*Reviews and general articles)

1. Watson JMG, Junger G, *Principles and Practice of Screening for Disease*. WHO Public Health Paper 34, 1968.
2. Greegor DH, Diagnosis of large-bowel cancer in the asymptomatic patient. *JAMA* 1967; **201**: 943–5.
3. Rozen P, The OMED Colorectal Cancer Screening Committee: a report of its aims and activities. *Gastrointest Endosc* 1999; **50**: 449–54.
4. Weller D, Hiller J, Beilby J, Woodward A, Screening for colorectal cancer. Knowledge, attitudes and practices of South Australian GPs. *Med J Aust* 1994; **160**: 620–4.
5. Winawer SJ, Fletcher RH, Miller L et al, Colorectal cancer screening: clinical guidelines and rationale. *Gastroenterology* 1997; **112**: 594–642.
6. *Young GP, Screening for colorectal cancer: an introduction. In: *Prevention and Early Detection of Colorectal Cancer* (Young GP, Rozen P, Levin B, eds). London: Saunders, 1996: 271–4.
7. Austoker J, Gaining informed consent for screening. *BMJ* 1999; **319**: 722–3.
8. Bini EJ, Rajapaksa RC, Weinshel EH, The findings and impact of nonrehydrated guaiac examination of the rectum (FINGER) study: a comparison of 2 methods of screening for colorectal cancer in asymptomatic average-risk patients. *Arch Intern Med* 1999; **159**: 2022–6.
9. Young GP, St John DJB. Selecting an occult blood test for use as a screening tool for large bowel cancer. *Front Gastrointest Res* 1991; **18**: 135–56.
10. Young GP, St John DJB, Winawer SJ, Rozen P, and the combined WHO/OMED FOBT Screening Committee, Choice of fecal occult blood tests for screening: recommendations based on performance characteristics in population studies. Submitted.
11. Young GP, Macrae FA, St John DJB. Clinical methods of early detection: basis, use and evaluation. In: *Prevention and Early Detection of Colorectal Cancer* (Young GP, Rozen P, Levin B, eds). London: Saunders, 1996: 241–70.
12. Petty MT, Deacon MC, Alexeyeff MA et al, Readability and sensitivity of a new faecal occult blood test in a hospital ward environment. *Med J Aust* 1992; **156**: 420–3.
13. *Sinatra M, St John DJB, Young GP, Interference of plant peroxidases with guaiac-based fecal occult blood tests is avoidable. *Clin Chem* 1999; **45**: 123–6.
14. Saito H, Yoshida Y, Mass screening: Japanese perspective. In: *Prevention and Early Detection of Colorectal Cancer* (Young GP, Rozen P, Levin B, eds). London: Saunders, 1996: 301–11.
15. Pierson RN, Holt PR, Watson RM, Keating RP, Aspirin and gastrointestinal bleeding. *Am J Med* 1961; **31**: 259–65.
16. Macrae FA, St John DJB, Relationship between patterns of bleeding and Hemoccult sensitivity in patients with colorectal cancers or adenomas. *Gastroenterology* 1982; **82**: 891–8.
17. *Rozen P, Knaani J, Samuel Z, Comparative screening with a sensitive guaiac and specific immunochemical occult blood test within an endoscopy study. *Cancer* 2000; **89**: 46–52.
18. Ferrucci JT, Screening for colon cancer: programs of the American College of Radiology. *Am J Radiol* 1993; **160**: 999–1003.
19. *Bampton PA, Young GP, Screening for colorectal cancer: use of colonoscopy or barium enema. *Semin Colon Rectal Surg* 2000; **11**: 9–15.

20. Winawer SJ, Stewart ET, Zauber AG et al, A comparison of colonoscopy and double-contrast barium enema for surveillance after polypectomy. *N Engl J Med* 2000; **342**: 1766–72.

21. *Selby JV, Friedman GD, Quesenberry CP Jr, Weiss NS, A case–control study of screening sigmoidoscopy and mortality from colorectal cancer. *N Engl J Med* 1992; **326**: 653–7.

22. Austoker J, Cancer prevention: setting the scene. *BMJ* 1994; **308**: 1415–20.

23. DATTA, Rigid and flexible sigmoidoscopies. *JAMA* 1990; **264**: 89–92.

24. Schapiro M, Lehman GA, *Flexible Sigmoidoscopy: Techniques and Utilization*. Baltimore: Williams & Wilkins, 1990.

25. Lieberman D, How to screen for colon cancer. *Annu Rev Med* 1998; **49**: 163–72.

26. *Lieberman DA, Weiss DG, Bond JH et al, Use of colonoscopy to screen asymptomatic adults for colorectal cancer. *N Engl J Med* 2000; **343**: 162–8.

27. American Society for Gastrointestinal Endoscopy. Endoscopy by non-physicians: guidelines for clinical application. *Gastrointest Endosc* 1999; **49**: 826–8.

28. American Society for Gastrointestinal Endoscopy, Guidelines for training non-specialists in in screening flexible sigmoidoscopy. *Gastrointest Endosc* 2000; **51**: 783–5.

29. Rex DK, Johnson DA, Lieberman DA et al, Colorectal cancer prevention 2000: screening recommendations of the American College of Gastroenterology. *Am J Gastroenterol* 2000; **95**: 868–77.

30. *Atkin WS, Morson BC, Cuzick J, Long-term risk of colorectal cancer after excision of rectosigmoid adenomas. *N Engl J Med* 1992; **326**: 658–62.

31. Irwig L, Glasziou P, Informed consent for screening by community sampling. *Eff Clin Pract* 2000; **3**: 47–50.

32. Macrae FA, Tan KG, Williams CB, Towards safer colonoscopy: a report on the complications of 5000 diagnostic or therapeutic colonoscopies. *Gut* 1983; **24**: 376–83.

33. Mandel JS, Bond JH, Church TR et al, Reducing mortality from colorectal cancer by screening for fecal occult blood. Minnesota Colon Cancer Control Study. *N Engl J Med* 1993; **328**: 1365–71.

34. Hardcastle JD, Chamberlain JO, Robinson MHE et al, Randomised controlled trial of faecal occult blood screening for colorectal cancer. *Lancet* 1996; **348**: 1472–7.

35. Kronborg O, Fenger C, Olsen J et al, Randomised study of screening for colorectal cancer with faecal occult blood test. *Lancet* 1996; **348**: 1467–71.

36. Mandel JS, Church TR, Bond JH et al, The effect of fecal occult-blood screening on the incidence of colorectal cancer. *N Engl J Med* 2000; **343**: 1603–7.

37. Olynyk JK, Aquilia S, Fletcher DR, Dickinson JA, Flexible sigmoidoscopy screening for colorectal cancer in average risk subjects: a community-based pilot project. *Med J Aust* 1996; **165**: 74–6.

38. Atkin WS, Hart A, Edwards R et al, Uptake, yield of neoplasia, and adverse effects of flexible sigmoidoscopy screening. *Gut* 1998; **42**: 560–5.

39. Rex DK, Lehman GA, Hawes RH et al, Screening colonoscopy in asymptomatic average-risk persons with negative fecal occult blood tests. *Gastroenterology* 1991; **100**: 64–7.

40. *Young GP, Screening for colorectal cancer: alternative fecal occult blood tests. *Eur J Gastroenterol Hepatol* 1998; **10**: 205–12.

41. Allison JE, Tekewa JS, Ransom LJ, Adrian AL, A comparison of fecal occult blood tests for colorectal cancer screening. *N Engl J Med* 1996; **334**: 144–59.

42. Newcomb PA, Norfleet RG, Storer BE et al, Screening sigmoidoscopy and colorectal cancer mortality. *J Natl Cancer Inst* 1992; **84**: 1572–5.

43. Neugut AI, Pita S, Role of sigmoidoscopy in screening for colorectal cancer: a critical review. *Gastroenterology* 1988; **95**: 492–9.

44. Selby JV, Targeting colonoscopy. *Gastroenterology* 1994; **106**: 1702–5.

45. Cotton PB, Williams CB, *Practical gastrointestinal endoscopy*. London: Blackwell Science, 1990.

46. Salkeld S, Young G, Irwig L et al, Cost-effectiveness analysis of screening by faecal occult blood testing for colorectal cancer in Australia. *Aust J Public Health* 1996; **20**: 138–43.

47. Taylor T, Williamson S, Wardle J et al, Acceptability of flexible sigmoidoscopy screening in older adults in the United Kingdom. *J Med Screen* 2000; **7**: 38–45.

48. *Wagner JL, Tunis S, Brown M et al, The cost-effectiveness of colorectal cancer screening in average-risk adults. In: *Prevention and Early Detection of Colorectal Cancer* (Young GP, Rozen P, Levin B, eds). London: Saunders, 1996: 321–56.

49. Umetani M, Sasaki S, Masaki T et al, Involvement of APC and K-ras mutation in non-polypoid colorectal tumorigenesis. *Br J Cancer* 2000; **81**: 9–15.

9 When colorectal cancer is detected, what treatment should follow?

Bernard Levin, John Skibber, Paul Rozen, Graeme P Young

Primary treatment of colorectal cancer

While the primary treatment of colorectal carcinoma must rely heavily on expert surgical resection, the comprehensive care of the patient with colorectal neoplasia requires a multidisciplinary approach. The need for adjuvant systemic chemotherapy or immunotherapy, with or without concurrent radiation therapy, depends on tumor location (colon versus rectum) and stage of disease. Systemic chemotherapy may also be indicated in those with metastatic colorectal cancer. Other supportive medical and nursing services are often required.

Surgical principles of management

Adenomas that contain adenocarcinomas

Since adenomatous polyps represent a spectrum of abnormalities between normal mucosa and invasive colorectal carcinoma, it is important to accurately determine the presence of tumor invasion in a colorectal adenoma that contains adenocarcinoma. Invasion through the muscularis mucosae and into the submucosa indicates the ability to spread through lymphatics and blood vessels.

Lesions in which carcinoma cells extend through the muscularis mucosae require complete excision and accurate assessment of the histology. The depth of invasion, degree of differentiation, adequacy of excision margins, and presence or absence of lymphatic or vascular invasion are all important characteristics that need to be assessed in an adenoma that contains adenocarcinoma. Adenomatous polyps may be either sessile or pedunculated. Invasive cancer occurs in about 10% of sessile polyps and 4.5% of pedunculated polyps, and overall about 3–5% of colorectal polyps contain invasive cancer.[1,2] Sessile polyps that have been removed in a piecemeal fashion usually cannot be properly staged. In the case of pedunculated polyps, when invasion does not extend into the base of the stalk, endoscopic removal is adequate treatment. Haggitt et al[3] studied a series of patients in whom colorectal cancers arose in adenomatous polyps with only minimal invasion of the colonic wall (Figure 9.1). They created a staging system for the depth of penetration into the stalk or base of the polyp that was correlated with outcomes. Polyps treated by piecemeal excision or those inadequately oriented are difficult to assess using this system. Level 1 tumors invade into the muscularis mucosae but are limited to the head of the polyp; level 2 carcinomas invade into the neck of the adenoma, and level 3 lesions invade into the stalk; level 4 indicates invasion into the submucosa of the bowel wall below the polyp but above the muscularis propria. Level 4 invasion signifies a T1 carcinoma. In the 65 patients of the study with only carcinoma in situ, there were no recurrences or carcinoma in lymph nodes at the time of colectomy. The group with pedunculated polyps where the carcinoma invaded only into the head of the polyp also had no adverse outcomes after endoscopic polypectomy (Table 9.1). These criteria have been confirmed in other series.[2,4]

Table 9.1 Risk factors for adverse outcome in patients with an adenoma that contains adenocarcinoma

	Low risk	High risk
Degree of differentiation	Good or moderate	Poor
Polypectomy margin	Clear or >2 mm	Involved by cancer
Venous or lymphatic invasion	Absent	Present
Invasion of submucosal bowel wall	Absent	Present

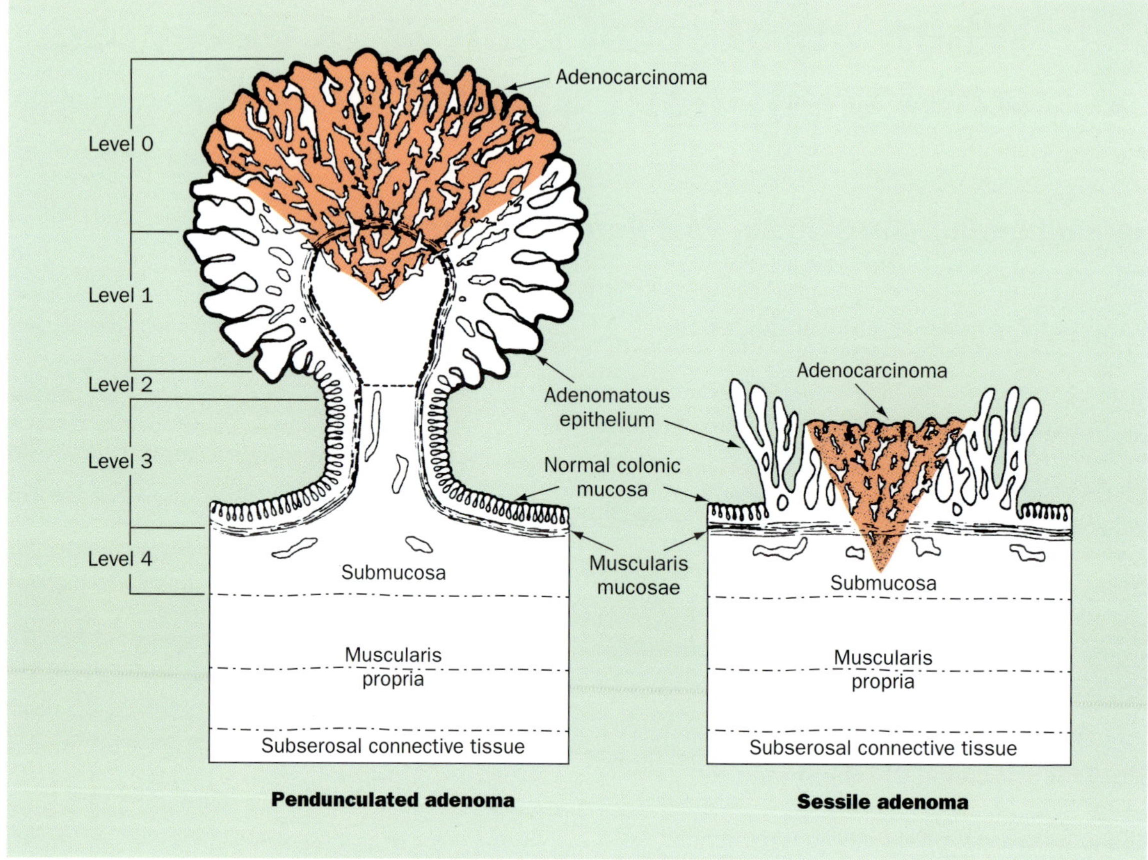

Figure 9.1 *Grading of neoplasia arising in an adenomatous polyp. From reference 3, with permission from WB Saunders.*

Ultimately, the decision to undertake a surgical resection in a patient with an adenoma that contains adenocarcinoma takes into account the gross and histologic pathology, the location of the lesion, the presence of comorbid disease, and the patient's wishes for treatment.

Relationship between stage of cancer and survival

The principles of staging of colorectal cancer are important, since there is a correlation between stage at diagnosis and survival.

In Table 9.2, the TNM classification used by the American Joint Committee on Cancer and the Union Internationale Contre le Cancer (UICC) is shown, together with a graphical demonstration of the T classification in Figure 9.2.[5] The relationship of stage to survival is indicated in Table 9.3.

Colon cancer resection: principles

The preoperative *evaluation* for resection of colon carcinoma includes an assessment of the patient's fitness for surgery and of the extent of spread of the tumor. Evaluation for synchronous colonic neoplasia by colonoscopy is important because of a 3–5% risk of having another cancer and a 30–40% incidence of adenomatous polyps. However, one cannot perform a preoperative evaluation of the entire colon in patients with obstructive lesions or in those who must have emergency surgery (e.g. for perforation), and postoperative evaluation of the colon will be required in such patients.

Surgical *resection* with an anastomosis is the treatment of choice in over 85% of patients with colon cancer. The majority of resections carried out for colon carcinoma are done with curative intent, even though some patients may have microscopic metastases that are undetectable at the time of laparotomy. During the surgical procedure, information is gained about the presence of visceral metastases and lymph node involvement. In performing a curative resection, the segment of colon bearing the primary tumor is first resected with adequate margins of normal-appearing tissue together with its major vascular pedicle and parallel lymphatic drainage, and an anastomosis is then performed (Figure 9.3).

Table 9.2 *The TNM classification according to the American Joint Committee on Cancer (AJCC) and the Union Internationale Contre le Cancer (UICC)[a]*

Tx	Minimum requirements to assess the primary tumor cannot be met
T0	No evidence of primary tumor
Tis	In situ carcinoma
T1	Tumor extends into the submucosa
T2	Tumor extends into the muscularis propria
T3	Tumor extends through the muscularis propria into the subserosa or into the non-peritonealized pericolic or perirectal tissues
T4	Tumor extends directly into other organs or tissues, or tumor perforates the visceral peritoneum of the specimen
Nx	Minimum requirements to assess the regional lymph nodes cannot be met
N0	No lymph node metastasis
N1	Metastatic tumor in one to three pericolic or perirectal lymph nodes
N2	Metastatic tumor in four or more pericolic or perirectal lymph nodes
N3	Metastatic to any lymph node along the course of a major named vascular trunk
Mx	Minimum requirements to assess distant metastasis cannot be met
M0	No distant metastasis
M1	Distant metastasis present

[a] Reproduced from reference 5, with permission from McGraw-Hill.

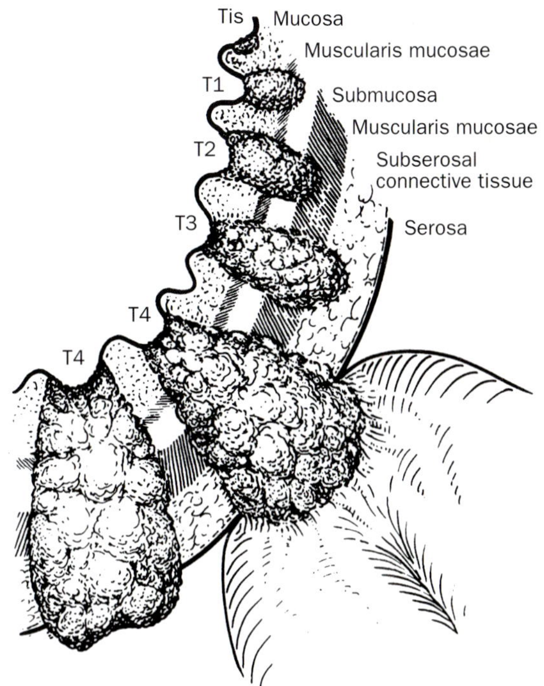

Figure 9.2 *Schematic demonstration of the TNM classification. Reproduced from reference 5 with permission from McGraw-Hill.*

Table 9.3 *Classification of large-bowel cancer by its degree of spread (stage, TNM features) and its correlation with survival[a]*

Stage groupings	TNM classification	5-year survival rate (%)
Stage 0	Tis, N0, M0	100
Stage I	T1, N0, M0	100
	T2, N0, M0	85
Stage II	T3, N0, M0	70
	T4, N0, M0	30
Stage III	Any T, N1, M0	60
	Any T, N2, M0	
	Any T, N3, M0	30
Stage IV	Any T, any N, M1	3

[a] Reproduced from reference 5, with permission from McGraw-Hill.

For *palliative* purposes, to relieve the symptoms of obstruction or bleeding, a more limited resection may be performed. In certain select circumstances, such as very advanced carcinomatosis, or in the presence of extensive tumors that invade the retroperitoneum or adjacent organs, simple diversion and colostomy, or bypass surgery, may be an alternative. By managing bleeding, obstruction, fistula formation, and perforation, surgical resection provides palliation.

In carcinoma of the *proximal half of the colon*, the distal 10–15 cm of ileum is resected together with the right half of the colon. This includes the related blood vessels and lymph nodes up to the base of the ileocolic artery. After transection of the distal ileum and the midtransverse colon, an anastomosis is then created (Figure 9.3). In tumors of the *transverse colon*, essentially the same operation can be performed, with an extension of the resection margin to the left of the middle colic arcade and inclusion of this arcade with the specimen. For lesions in the *left colon*, left colectomy involves a resection of the bowel supplied by the inferior mesenteric artery, and anastomosis is done between the distal transverse colon and rectum. In carcinomas of the *sigmoid colon*, a similar operation is performed to that for left colon carcinoma. When an *obstructing* lesion or *synchronous lesions* are present in the left colon, a total abdominal colectomy may be performed, with an anastomosis between the terminal ileum and the rectum. Most commonly,

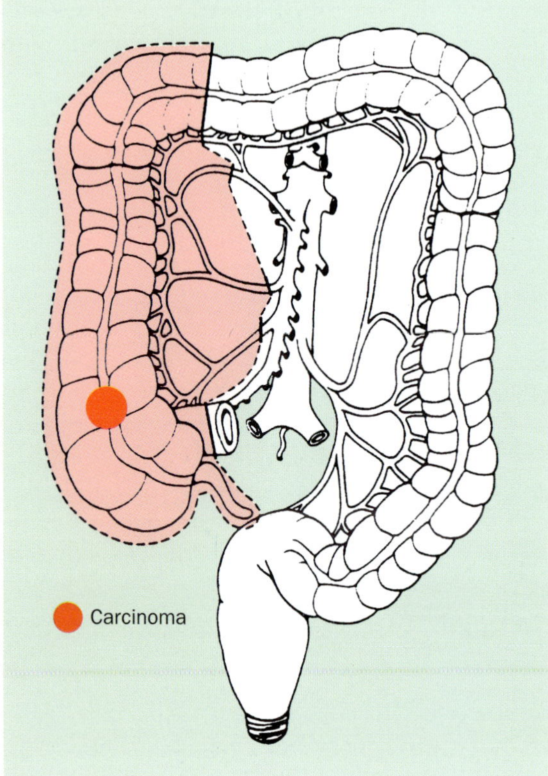

Figure 9.3 *Demonstrating principles of resection for colon cancer: (1) resection with wide luminal margins; (2) lymphadenectomy by mesenteric resection to include the major arterial vessels supplying the affected segment; (3) reconstruction by primary anastomosis.*

perforated tumors adhere to adjacent organs, and should be resected en bloc with any adherent organs. Free perforation causes peritonitis, and should be managed urgently by resection of the perforated segment.

Postoperatively, the most troublesome complications are bleeding and anastomotic leaks. While bleeding manifests itself during or immediately after the operation, anastomotic leaks usually occur 3–7 days after surgery. Fever, leukocytosis, abdominal pain, and prolonged ileus may occur as a result, and signs of systemic sepsis may supervene. In leaks that are walled off, a fistula may develop. Computed tomography (CT) scan is often helpful in identifying abscesses due to anastomotic leaks. Percutaneous drainage may occasionally be useful in managing this complication, but most patients require reoperation.

Laparoscopic colectomy

Laparoscopic colectomy for colon cancer can be performed safely by the experienced abdominal surgeon, although there is a significant 'learning curve'. More rapid recovery and less pain from the procedure occur in many patients. The oncologic safety of the procedure is still unproven, and it remains to be determined whether recurrence and survival are comparable to those who undergo a conventional colectomy. The occasional reports of isolated port-site cancer recurrences are also of concern.

Rectal cancer resection: principles

In rectal cancer, treatment decisions are based on accurate preoperative clinical and radiologic staging. The extent of tumor spread locally and distantly greatly affects treatment planning. Endorectal ultrasound is a useful and accurate technique for determining the depth of penetration of the bowel wall by primary rectal tumors (Figure 9.4).

The principles of resection for rectal cancer involve removal of the tumor with normal tissue margins, the assessment of lymph node involvement, and the restoration of function. Owing to the anatomic location of the rectum in the pelvis and the tendency for lateral spread of these tumors, local recurrence rates are higher than in colon cancer. In addition, the presence of a low rectal cancer may limit the ability to excise a lesion while preserving the anus, thus making a colostomy likely.

Local excision for rectal cancer

Transrectal full-thickness local excision is an effective treatment of selected early low rectal cancers. Local excision is used as curative therapy for patients who have a superficial tumor and as alternative therapy in medically compromised patients and those who refuse standard therapy.

The intent of local excision is to be technically feasible and obtain a negative-margin full-thickness excision and a

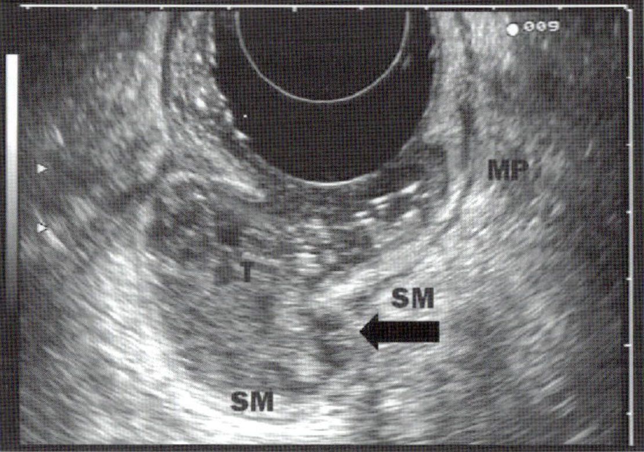

Figure 9.4 *Endorectal ultrasonogram of a T2 rectal adenocarcinoma demonstrating depth of tumor invasion. SM, submucosa; MP, muscularis propria; arrow, tumor invading submucosa. (Figure provided by Dr M Santo, Tel Aviv.)*

low risk of there being lymph node metastases. Physical assessment, CT, and endorectal ultrasound are helpful in the preoperative evaluation of rectal cancer patients. Imaging findings can be used to select patients for local excision procedures by determining the depth of tumor penetration into the rectal wall and the absence of enlarged lymph nodes. Most patients with rectal cancer do not meet the criteria for treatment by local excision alone because of the size or extent of the tumor spread. Curative surgical treatment for rectal cancer entails tumor excision with margins of normal tissue and resection of locoregional lymph nodes, whereas local excision alone achieves a negative-margin excision without resection of the mesorectal lymph nodes.

The incidence of lymph node metastases in patients with T1 tumors approximates the recurrence rate for T1 cancers treated by local excision, which is a 3–10% rate of local recurrence.[6] Survival rates in patients with T1 rectal carcinomas treated by local excision or radical resection are 90–100%.[7] Local excision is a reasonable treatment for T1 carcinoma of the rectum if favorable criteria are present. Poor differentiation and perineural, blood vessel, or lymphatic invasion are significant predictors of lymph node involvement and poor survival. In such cases, standard surgical therapy should be used. If the patient refuses or cannot tolerate standard surgical therapy, the use of adjuvant therapy after local excision should be considered.

The risk of lymph node metastasis is 10–30% in patients with T2 rectal carcinoma.[8,9] Studies show higher local recurrence rates for tumors involving the muscularis propria treated by local excision, because of the failure to treat lymphatic metastases. Recurrence rates are 17–24% in patients with T2 tumors, and survival rates are 78–82% in those treated by local excision. In patients with T2 carcinomas of the rectum, the risk of lymph node metastasis in the mesorectum must be addressed by resection of the mesorectum during proctectomy or, if a local excision is performed, by the addition of chemotherapy and radiation therapy to reduce the incidence of pelvic recurrence. Excellent disease control rates are possible for patients with selected T1 and T2 rectal cancers treated by local excision and postoperative adjuvant radiotherapy[10] (Table 9.4). In contrast, local excision cannot be recommended for T3 rectal cancer.

Locoregional resection and multimodality treatment for rectal cancer

About 60–80% of patients with rectal cancer have stage II or stage III lesions that are frequently large and biologically aggressive. They are at higher risk of local and systemic recurrence after treatment. The risk of spread to local lymph nodes and of local recurrence increases as tumor penetration of the rectal wall deepens. This has led to the development of surgical procedures, such as abdominoperineal resection, that can achieve tumor-free proximal and distal tissue margins and remove the proximal pathways of lymphatic spread from rectal cancer. A distal margin of 2 cm from the edge of the tumor has been shown to be adequate. However, the work of Quirke and colleagues has demonstrated the importance of lateral tumor spread in influencing local recurrence of rectal cancer after resection.[11–13]

The bony sidewalls of the pelvis confine the rectum together with major blood vessels and nerves, and the pelvis contains viscera that are important to functional well-being. These anatomical characteristics do not facilitate obtaining wide margins of normal tissue around a transmural rectal tumor. Tumor involvement at the circumferential margin of resection is associated with local recurrence in 85% of cases,[10] with a resulting poor prognosis[12,13] (Figure 9.5). While distal margins are measured in centimeters, circumferential margins are measured in millimeters. Controlled sharp dissection must be done with close attention to these margins. Involvement of the circumferential margins can be due to direct spread, mesenteric implants, vascular or lymphatic invasion, or cancer-bearing lymph nodes.[11] Tumor involvement of the circumferential margins of resection is frequently due to

Table 9.4 *Patterns of failure by American Joint Commission on Cancer tumor (T) stage of disease after local excision and adjuvant therapy for rectal cancer[a]*

	T1 (*n* =16)	T2 (*n* =15)	T3 (*n* =15)	Total (*n* =46)
Local recurrence only	0	0	2	2 (4%)
Distant recurrence only	0	0	4	4 (7%)
Combined recurrence	0	1	1	2 (4%)

[a] Reproduced from reference 10, with permission from WB Saunders.

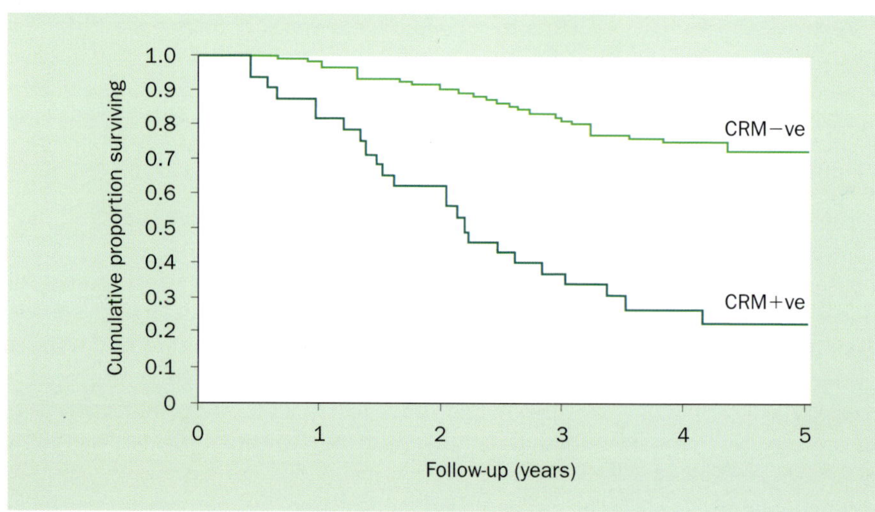

Figure 9.5 *Survival comparing presence or absence of tumor at the circumferential resection margin (CRM) in patients who underwent potentially curative resection. Derived from reference 13, with permission from the* Lancet.

spread in the mesorectum distal to the primary tumor.[12] The mesorectum is the extension of the large-bowel mesentery along the posterior wall of the rectum. This blood-vessel- and lymph-node-bearing structure is enveloped by the fascia propria of the rectum. Total mesorectal excision has been demonstrated to be effective in the surgical management of rectal cancer. Consequently, there is much interest in the use of surgery alone for node-negative T2 and T3 rectal cancer when optimal surgical techniques such as total mesorectal excision and sharp dissection are used.[14]

For rectal cancer patients, a major component of quality of life is sphincter preservation. This is simple to accomplish in middle and upper rectal cancers, for which low anterior resection allows adequate removal of the tumor and surrounding lymphatics and an end-to-end anastomosis. In patients with low rectal cancers that do not involve the levator muscles or sphincters, the anus may still be spared by proctectomy and coloanal anastomosis. Preoperative chemoradiation may facilitate this goal.[15] However, patients with levator ani or sphincter involvement are best managed by abdominoperineal resection and permanent colostomy.

Proctectomy and coloanal anastomosis can be useful in patients with low rectal cancer,[16] as demonstrated in a study in which the median distance of the tumor from the anal verge was 6–7 cm. The operation required complete mobilization of the rectum to the levators, transanal transection of the rectum, complete mobilization of the left colon, and endoanal anastomosis. The effectiveness of the procedure was demonstrated by a relatively low local recurrence rate of 7%. Fecal continence was satisfactory in 78% of patients, and overall bowel function appeared to be improved in patients who had a colonic J-pouch reservoir

created with a coloanal anastomosis (Figure 9.6). Early and late complications were related to anastomotic leakage (10%) and stricture formation. Major long-term postoperative complaints are related to diminished rectal capacity. This function gradually improves over an approximately 9-month period after closure of the temporary stoma.

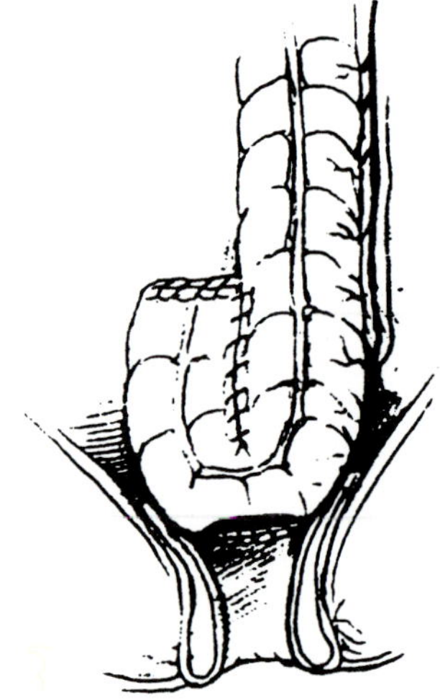

Figure 9.6 *Coloanal anastomosis is defined as a method of restoring bowel continuity by uniting the descending colon to the anal canal. It is in wide use in the management of cancers of the middle and lower thirds of the rectum. A detailed anal continence history and physical examination by an experienced surgeon are very important in predicting the postoperative outcome. Functional results of a 'straight' coloanal anastomosis, especially increased frequency, have led to the preference for use of a J-pouch. This has the functional consequence of creating a reservoir for fecal contents.*

Considerable tumor reduction can occur after preoperative radiation or chemoradiation. With radiation alone, the complete pathologic response rate of lesions that have infiltrated through the bowel wall and/or have involved local lymph nodes is reported to be 10–17%. With preoperative chemoradiation, complete response rates can be increased to 20–30%[17-21] (Table 9.5). In a patient with a locally advanced primary rectal cancer or in the presence of pelvic recurrence, an extensive surgical procedure is often needed to provide clear margins. Preoperative chemoradiation is frequently used for such tumors, especially if they appear fixed.[22] An increased resectability rate can be achieved without an increase in morbidity.[23-25] Perineal reconstructive procedures are often required to manage the pelvic defect.[26] The majority of local recurrences from rectal cancer are unresectable owing to a variety of factors, and palliative measures, including stent placement or laser photoablation, may be indicated.

Surgical management of hepatic metastases

Fifteen percent of patients will have metastases to the liver at the time of presentation with the primary tumor. Failure of curative treatment for colorectal cancer will be frequently manifested by the occurrence of hepatic metastases, and in about 30% of patients, the liver will be the only site of metastatic disease at the time of death from colorectal cancer.[27]

Untreated, hepatic metastases will generally result in a median survival of less than 2 years.[28] The length of survival is influenced by the extent of hepatic disease, the presence of extrahepatic metastases or an unresected primary, and the severity of comorbid disease. About 60% of patients who present with a solitary liver metastasis will survive over 1 year even if untreated, while only 5% of patients with widespread disease will survive more than 1 year. While unresected hepatic metastases will cause death in almost all patients within 5 years of diagnosis, it has been demonstrated that hepatic resection in appropriately selected patients can result in a survival rate of approximately 25–30% at 5 years, with a median survival of 28–35 months.[29,30] However, only highly selected patients will benefit from a surgical approach to apparently isolated hepatic metastases.

The majority of patients found to have hepatic metastases during follow-up after curative therapy will have these discovered by a CT scan (Figure 9.7) whose performance was prompted by a rising carcinoembryonic antigen (CEA) level, abdominal pain, or jaundice. About 80% of patients with hepatic metastases will have elevated CEA levels. A multiphase helical abdominal CT scan can determine the extent of hepatic metastases, and identify extrahepatic metastases. Abdominal ultrasound is less sensitive, and is not useful for determining resectability. Additional procedures to determine the extent of disease in patients found to have hepatic metastases are chest CT scan and colonoscopy. The exclusion of extrahepatic disease

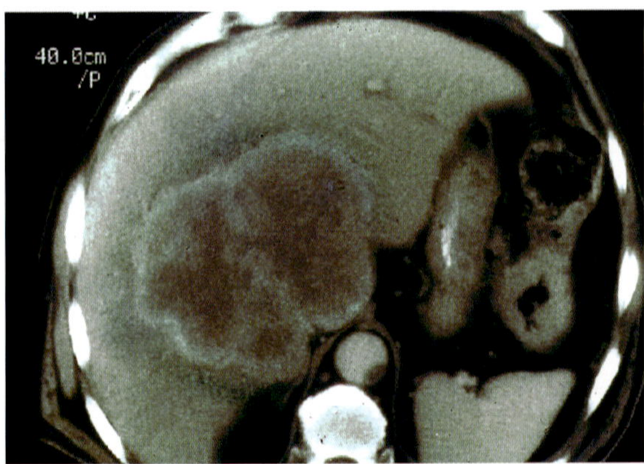

Figure 9.7 *CT scan demonstrating multiple hepatic metastases.*

Table 9.5 *Correlation of rectal cancer response to preoperative oncological regimen*

Study[a]	No. of patients	Preoperative EBRT[b] dose (Gy)	Chemotherapy[c]	Complete response rate (%)
University of Florida[17]	132	30–50	None	11
Jewish Hospital[18]	208	40–50	None	6
MDACC[19]	77	45	5-FU infusion	29
Duke University[21]	43	45	5-FU + cisplatin	27
MSKCC[21]	20	50.4	5-FU + leucovorin	20

[a] MDACC, MD Anderson Cancer Center; MSKCC, Memorial Sloan-Kettering Cancer Center.
[b] EBRT, external-beam radiation therapy. [c] 5-FU, 5-fluorouracil.

is critical to the selection of patients for hepatic resection. Hepatic arteriography is used to evaluate the hepatic arterial anatomy or to plan for placement of an hepatic arterial infusion pump for liver-directed chemotherapy.[31]

Hepatic resection: principles

To be successful, hepatic resection must accomplish complete removal of the tumor with adequate margins of normal tissue. Usually, margins of approximately 1 cm are obtained. The major limitation to wider resection margins within the liver is the relationship of the tumor to major vascular structures within or adjacent to the liver, including the vena cava or hepatic veins, the portal vein, or the hepatic arteries. Recognition of intrahepatic structures can be greatly enhanced by intraoperative ultrasound, and tumors as small as 5 mm can be identified. At times, ultrasound techniques can be also useful in guiding fine-needle aspiration of suspicious lesions. At the time of laparotomy, the surgeon performs a thorough exploration for extrahepatic spread before attempting hepatic tumor resection.

Hepatic resections are broadly defined as either anatomic or non-anatomic.[32] Non-anatomic resections are also known as segmental resections. Anatomic resections are usually termed right and left lobectomy, lateral segmentectomy, and trisegmentectomy.[30] Anatomic resection is not necessary for small lesions in a favorable location. The benefit of non-anatomic resection is that it limits the amount of functional hepatic parenchyma that is removed, thereby diminishing postoperative hepatic insufficiency. Non-anatomic resections have also been shown to decrease blood loss and shorten operating room times and hospital stays.[33] For larger tumors and those located adjacent to major portal or hepatic vein branches, anatomic resection is usually preferable. The mortality rate associated with hepatic resection for colorectal metastases is 5% or less, with the majority of deaths being due to hemorrhage, infection, liver failure, or biliary leaks.[30,32] Among those whose cancer recurs, the liver is the most likely site of recurrence.

Because the majority of patients with hepatic metastases are not candidates for hepatic resection, other regional treatment measures include cryoablation of the hepatic tumor with a margin of surrounding hepatic parenchyma.[34] Another type of treatment is hepatic arterial chemotherapy, which is based not only on the selective vascular supply of hepatic metastases from the arterial blood flow but also on the high hepatic extraction of certain chemotherapeutic agents such as floxuridine.[35] While hepatic arterial pump placement may be associated with many technical complications, including arterial thrombosis or catheter dislodgement, intra-arterial therapy does provide a high degree of tumor shrinkage in the liver. A major drawback to this treatment, however, is that metastatic disease may develop at extrahepatic sites during treatment. The overall impact on patient survival is modest.

Lung metastasis

The management of lung metastases follows similar principles of management to those for hepatic metastasis. In the absence of other sites of metastatic disease, a solitary lung metastasis may be resected with reasonable results. However, the majority of patients have extensive recurrence that is more appropriately treated with systemic chemotherapy.

Patterns of failure

As a basis for selecting additional therapy, it is important to understand where colorectal cancer spreads after attempted curative resection. Approximately 75% of all patients with colorectal cancer will present at a stage when all gross carcinoma can be surgically resected. The natural history and patterns of failure (local recurrence or distal spread) following apparently 'curative' resection, differ for colon and rectal cancer. Locoregional failure, as the only or major site of recurrence, is more common in rectal cancer, although lung metastases are well described. The rationale for a locally effective therapy in rectal cancer, such as pelvic irradiation, is based on this natural history. Colon cancer frequently spreads to the liver, peritoneum, and other distant sites, and is associated with a lower rate of local failure.

Adjuvant therapy of colon cancer

Despite an apparently high rate of surgical resectability, about half of all patients with colorectal cancer die from metastatic disease. In particular, those with locally advanced tumors (transmucosal spread or with lymph node involvement) may have subclinical micrometastases. Viable tumor cells may have metastasized prior to primary tumor resection. They may be in the adjacent lymph nodes or bone marrow but not detectable except by special histological or molecular techniques. This realization led to the use of adjuvant cytotoxic therapy administered with intent to cure. The target of such therapy is the pool of rapidly cycling cancer cells that may be circulating. The aim is to eradicate them before they become established and relatively refractory to treatment. Postoperative adjuvant therapy after surgery is advised for most patients with stage III colon cancer, and this is based on the recommendations of the 1990 US National Institutes of Health (NIH) consensus statement as well as subsequent trials.[36–38] A clear advantage of such therapy for those with stage II cancer is being evaluated, but has not been demonstrated yet.

For approximately 40 years, the only drug to show reproducible therapeutic activity in colorectal cancer was 5-fluorouracil (5-FU). 5-FU is believed to act mainly by intracellular conversion to the corresponding deoxyriboside monophosphate, 5-fluorodeoxyuridine monophosphate. This compound binds to and inhibits the enzyme thymidylate synthase, which is involved in the rate-limiting step in the de novo synthesis of thymidine nucleotides required for DNA synthesis. The compound leucovorin (folinic acid) modulates the activity of 5-FU, thereby enhancing therapeutic response rates compared with 5-FU alone. The results of recent trials in stage III colon cancer are summarized in Table 9.6. In the IMPACT analysis of three studies, mortality was reduced by 22%.[36] In an intergroup study in the USA, mortality was reduced by 16%.[37]

The currently popular regimens for the use of 5-FU plus leucovorin for adjuvant therapy for colon cancer include the following:

- a 'low-dose' leucovorin regimen consisting of leucovorin and 5-FU both administered by rapid intravenous injections daily for 5 consecutive days, with courses repeated every 4 weeks for 6 months;
- a 'high-dose' weekly leucovorin regimen consisting of 5-FU by rapid intravenous injection given at the 1-hour timepoint during a 2-hour infusion of leucovorin weekly for 6 weeks, with courses repeated every 8 weeks for 6 months.

The combination of 5-FU, leucovorin, and irinotecan (described below) is also likely to be incorporated into postoperative adjuvant therapy, based on the enhanced therapeutic activity of this combination in patients with metastatic colorectal cancer.

Immunotherapy

Immunotherapeutic approaches to the management of colorectal cancer have included trials of vaccines made from autologous tumor, tumor antigens produced by genetically engineered viruses, and anti-idiotype antibodies. Passive administration of monoclonal antibodies that recognize colorectal tumor antigens to patients with metastatic disease has failed to demonstrate clinical effectiveness. However, in an adjuvant trial involving patients with stage II and III colon and rectal cancer, intravenous administration of the murine monoclonal antibody 17-1A directed against a glycoprotein antigen commonly exposed on adenocarcinomas resulted in improved survival compared with surgery alone.[39] Confirmatory trials with monoclonal 17-1A in stage II colon cancer and in combination with 5-FU and leucovorin in stage III disease are in progress in North America and Europe.

Adjuvant therapy of rectal cancer

As surgical advances have reduced the need for abdominoperineal resection in the management of carcinoma of the rectum, adjuvant therapy has been shown to be valuable in reducing local and distant tumor recurrences. Local recurrence in the pelvis is often painful because of the involvement of contiguous organs and soft and bony tissues. Presenting symptoms vary from vague pelvic fullness to difficulty in voiding and sciatica. The effectiveness of postoperative irradiation and 5-FU-based chemotherapy as adjuvant therapy for resected high-risk rectal cancer (stage II or III disease) was established by prospective randomized trials during the 1980s and 1990s.[40–44] These and later trials are summarized in Table 9.7.[45]

Postoperative radiation therapy has been shown to reduce the risk of local recurrence but not to enhance overall survival in patients with stage II and III rectal cancer. Recently, the use of chemotherapy in combination with radiation therapy has been optimized in a study by the Gastrointestinal Intergroup in the USA that showed a reduction in the occurrence rate of distant metastases with improved relapse-free and overall survival for patients treated with continuous infusion of 5-FU.[44] A typical treatment regimen consists of 5-FU and leucovorin administered as a rapid intravenous infusion on days 1 and 5, on days 134–138, and on days 169–173. Patients receive a protracted infusion of 5-FU 225 mg/m^2/day by portable ambulatory infusion pump during the entire period of pelvic irradiation. Pelvic radiation therapy to the tumor bed and nodal groups begins on day 64 with a multiple-field technique. A total of 4500 cGy, in 180 cGy fractions, is administered over a 5-week period. Upon completion, patients receive a boost dose of 540 cGy to the entire tumor bed and adjacent lymph nodes.

Table 9.6 *Summary of recent trials comparing 5-fluorouracil/leucovorin (folinic acid) (5-FU/LV) against control in the adjuvant treatment of stage III colon cancer*

Trials (no. in study); randomized comparison; follow-up period	Disease-free survival rate (%)		Overall survival rate (%)	
	5-FU/LV	Control	5-FU/LV	Control
Overview of French, Italian, and Canadian trials ($n = 1493$);[36] 5-FU/HDLV versus observation;[a] 3 years	71	62[b]	83	78[c]
Intergroup study ($n = 309$);[37] 5-FU/LDLV versus observation;[a] 5 years	74	58[d]	74	63[e]

[a] HD, high dose; LD, low dose. [b] $p < 0.0001$; [c] $p = 0.03$; [d] $p < 0.004$; [e] $p = 0.02$.

Table 9.7 *Randomized postoperative chemoradiation trials in rectal cancer*[a]

Trial	Local failure rate (%)[b]	Distant failure rate (%)	Overall survival rate (%)
Gastrointestinal Tumor Study Group:			
Radiotherapy and chemotherapy	11	26	57
Radiotherapy	20	30	43
Chemotherapy	27	27	43
Control	24	34	28
National Surgical Adjuvant Breast and Bowel Program:			
Chemotherapy	21	24	58
Radiotherapy	16	31	50
Control	25	26	48
North Central Cancer Treatment Group:			
Radiotherapy and chemotherapy	14	29	53
Radiotherapy	25	46	38
Gastrointestinal Intergroup (USA):[c]			
Radiotherapy: PVI 5-FU	NS	31	70
Radiotherapy: bolus 5-FU	NS	40	60

[a] Modified from reference 45, with permission.
[b] NS, not studied.
[c] PVI, prolonged (peripheral) venous infusion; 5-FU, 5-fluorouracil.

Neoadjuvant therapy

Preoperative radiation therapy has been shown to reduce local tumor recurrence, but it has no impact on overall survival. The combination of chemotherapy and radiation therapy has resulted in higher rates of complete pathologic response compared with radiation therapy alone.[17–21] The acute complications of chemoradiation include diarrhea and tenesmus due to proctitis and increased frequency of urination due to bladder irritation. Chronically, radiation proctitis may result, with occasional bleeding. Rarely, small-bowel injury may be severe enough to result in obstruction due to stricture formation. These effects can be avoided by prone positioning techniques that move the small bowel out of the pelvis, and the use of bladder distention.

Management of advanced colorectal cancer

The patient with advanced colorectal cancer may present with local recurrence and/or widespread metastases. Characteristic sites of spread include the pelvis, retroperitoneum, liver, and lungs. The prognosis may vary considerably in each individual, depending on the extent of the disease and the presence of comorbid illnesses. A decision to offer chemotherapy or other treatment will depend upon the patient's general level of fitness (performance status), the extent of metastatic spread, and the wishes of the patient. Increasingly, because of access to the Internet, patients and their family members have more information concerning available treatment alternatives.

The management of advanced colorectal cancer requires appropriate integration of palliative measures such as chemotherapy and radiation therapy, as well as control of anorexia, fatigue, pain, and nausea. Mechanical bowel obstruction may require surgical decompression. Occasionally, depression and anxiety may be severe enough to warrant pharmacological therapy. The support of the medical oncologist and primary-care physician is especially crucial during this phase of the patient's illness.

Systemic chemotherapy

For over 40 years, the standard chemotherapeutic regimen for advanced (metastatic) colorectal cancer has been 5-FU, and, more recently, 5-FU modulated by leucovorin. Typical results obtained by the use of bolus 5-FU and leucovorin include partial response rates of 15–20% without clear evidence of a beneficial impact on survival for all those treated. However, palliation of symptoms may be achieved in responding patients. Alternative outpatient regimens have included continuous infusion of 5-FU using permanent venous access devices and portable infusion pumps. Typical temporary side-effects of 5-FU plus leucovorin therapy include nausea, vomiting, diarrhea, and oral stomatitis.

The oral chemotherapeutic agent UFT (a combination of tegafur and uracil) is the first of a new class of anti-cancer drugs called dihydropyrimidine dehydrogenase-inhibitory fluoropyrimidines. UFT combines uracil with the prodrug tegafur in a 4 : 1 molar ratio. Uracil completely inhibits the degradation of 5-FU, which results in a sustained concentration of 5-FU in tumor tissue. Trials conducted in the USA have demonstrated that this oral drug can be combined safely with leucovorin with similar efficacy to intravenous 5-FU and leucovorin.[46] Other new oral fluoropyrimidines such as capecitabine (Hoffmann-LaRoche) also have therapeutic activity in metastatic colon cancer.[47] Oral chemotherapeutic agents offer convenience and potential cost savings.

The topisomerase-1 inhibitor irinotecan (CPT-11) has been shown to benefit patients who are no longer responding to 5-FU therapy. Recently, the US Food and Drug Administration approved a new indication for irinotecan hydrochloride injection (Camptosar: Pharmacia and Upjohn Inc, Kalamazoo, MI) as first-line therapy in combination with 5-FU and leucovorin to treat metastatic colorectal cancer. The approval was based on the results of two multicenter, randomized controlled trials in Europe and the USA. In the European study, a statistically significant improvement in survival was observed (median 17.4 versus 14.1 months; $p < 0.005$) and in the US study, a statistically significant increase (median 14.8 versus 12.6 months ($p < 0.05$) was found.[48] Common side-effects include nausea, neutropenia, neutropenic fever, mucositis, and diarrhea.

Oxaliplatin (Sanofi-Synthelabo) is another new chemotherapeutic agent that has been used alone or in combination with 5-FU in patients whose tumors are resistant to 5-FU.[49] Oxaliplatin has not yet been approved for use in the USA, but is available in Europe and other countries. Trials of the combination of oxaliplatin and irinotecan are in progress.

For many patients, access to investigational therapy offers hope after conventional therapy has failed. These trials are accessible through major cancer centers in many countries or the Community Cooperative Oncology Group in the USA. Examples of new therapeutic approaches are summarized in Table 9.8. In the USA and possibly other Western countries, an estimated 50–60% of patients with cancer use complementary alternative medicine (CAM), and most of these patients combine CAM with conventional medicine. CAM may include herbal, biological, nutritional, chemical, or other interventions.[50]

Table 9.8 *New therapeutic approaches in advanced colorectal cancer*

- Growth antagonists: e.g. inhibitors of *ras* oncogene function
- Cancer vaccines
- Antiangiogenesis agents: e.g. anti-VEGF (vascular endothelial growth factor) antibody or inhibitors

Surveillance after colorectal cancer resection

The major aims of postoperative follow-up are the following:

- discover metastatic tumors at an early enough stage to permit definitive therapy;
- assess the results of surgical therapy and identify disease that requires further treatment;
- monitor patients for metachronous tumor development in the large bowel.

The value of such follow-up has been challenged because an estimated 17–61% of cancers may recur between scheduled return appointments and also because great expense is incurred by the use of radiological and laboratory tests, including CEA determinations.[51] In addition, one must consider the psychological distress caused by false-positive results, the possible failure of early detection, the discovery of asymptomatic, incurable recurrences, and the morbidity related to exploratory laparotomy done as a result of true-positive or false-positive results.

The most important time for follow-up is during the first 3 years after primary tumor resection. During this time, 85% of recurrences usually occur. Although there is still controversy about the most appropriate schedule of follow-up procedures, the following represents the practice of some physicians in the USA for relatively fit patients with stage I–III disease in whom further surgical or other therapies would be appropriate if recurrence were demonstrated:

- For the first 2 years, history and physical examination are performed every 6 months, as well as colonoscopy after the first year. CEA, CT of the abdomen and pelvis, and chest X-ray are performed at 6-month intervals, although the value of such examinations remains controversial in the asymptomatic patient.
- In the third year, history, physical examination, and CEA determination are performed every 6 months, and the time interval between CT scans is lengthened to 1 year. After the third year, patients are seen annually for history and physical examination.
- Colonoscopy is performed every 3 years after the first year if no abnormalities have been found. Flexible proctosigmoidoscopy is performed at 6- to 12-month intervals for the first 3 years in patients who have undergone a low anterior resection. However, it is worth noting that curable anastomatic recurrence is infrequent.[51]
- When an elevated CEA level is detected in a patient in whom it was normal postoperatively, the test should be repeated for confirmation. After confirmation, further evaluations may include imaging studies of the abdomen and chest, as well as colonoscopy. MRI, PET scans, and radioimmunoscintigraphy may be useful in this clinical situation.

Multidisciplinary approach to management

The optimal management of the patient with colorectal cancer requires a comprehensive and multidisciplinary approach involving the primary-care physician, surgeon, gastroenterologist, medical oncologist, radiation oncologist, pathologist, diagnostic radiologist, and specialized nurses (e.g. enterostomal therapists), as well as other support personnel.

Conclusions

The best outcome in the management of patients with colorectal neoplasia is achieved by detection of colorectal neoplasms at the earliest possible stage. The importance of screening and early detection cannot be overemphasized. The modern largely successful management of patients with stage I and II colorectal cancer rests heavily on the expertise of the surgeon, pathologist, and gastroenterologist. For patients with stage III and especially stage IV colorectal cancer, more effective management techniques are needed.

References (*Reviews and general articles)

1. Wolff WI, Shinya H, A new approach to colonic polyps. *Ann Surg* 1973; **178:** 367–76.
2. *Hamilton SR, Pathology and biology of colorectal neoplasia. In: *Prevention and Early Detection of Colorectal Cancer* (Young GP, Rozen P, Levin B, eds). London: Saunders, 1996: 3–21.
3. Haggitt RC, Glotzbach RE, Soffer EE, Wruble LD, Prognostic factors in colorectal carcinomas arising in adenomas: implications for lesions removed by endoscopic polypectomy. *Gastroenterology* 1985; **89:** 328–36.
4. *Volk EE, Goldblum JR, Petras RE et al, Management and outcome of patients with invasive carcinoma arising in colorectal polyps. *Gastroenterology* 1995; **109:** 1801–07.
5. *Fielding LP, Staging systems. In: *Cancer of the Colon, Rectum and Anus* (Cohen AM, Winawer SJ, Friedman MA, Gunderson LJ, eds). New York: McGraw-Hill, 1995: 207–15.
6. Graham RA, Gainsey L, Jessup JM, Local excision of rectal carcinoma. *Am J Surg* 1990; **160:** 306–12.
7. McDermott FT, Hughes ESR, Pihl E et al, Local recurrence after potentially curative resection for rectal cancer in a series of 1008 patients. *Br J Surg* 1985; **72:** 34–7.
8. Morson BC, Factors influencing the prognosis of early cancer of the rectum. *Br J Surg* 1966; **59:** 607–8.
9. *Minsky BD, Rich TA, Recht A et al. Selection criteria for local excision with or without adjuvant radiation therapy for rectal cancer. *Cancer* 1989; **63:** 1421–9.
10. Ota DM, Skibber JM, Rich TA, M. D. Anderson Cancer Center experience with local excision and multimodality therapy for rectal cancer. *Surg Clin North Am* 1992; **1:** 147–53.
11. Quirke P, Durdy P, Dixon MF et al. Local recurrence of rectal adenocarcinoma due to inadequate surgical resection: histopathological study of lateral tumor spread and surgical excision. *Lancet* 1986; **ii:** 996–9.
12. *Quirke P, Scott N, The pathologist's role in the assessment of local recurrence in rectal carcinoma. *Surg Oncol Clin North Am* 1992; **1:** 1–17.
13. Adam IJ, Mohamdee MO, Martin I et al, Role of circumferential involvement in the local recurrence of rectal cancer. *Lancet* 1994; **344:** 707–11.
14. McAnena OJ, Heald RI, Lockhart-Mummery HE, Operative and functional results of total mesorectal excision with ultra-low anterior resection in the management of carcinoma of the lower one-third of the rectum. *Surg Gynecol Obstet* 1990; **170:** 517–21.
15. Marks G, Mohuiddin M, Eitan A et al, High-dose preoperative radiation and radical-sphincter preserving surgery for rectal cancer. *Arch Surg* 1991; **126:** 1534–40.
16. Cavaliere F, Pemberton JH, Cosimelli M et al, Coloanal anastomosis for rectal cancer: long-term results at the Mayo and Cleveland Clinics. *Dis Colon Rectum* 1995; **38:** 807–12.
17. Mendenhall WM, Bland KI, Copeland EM et al, Does preoperative radiation therapy enhance the probability of local control and survival in high-risk distal rectal cancer? *Ann Surg* 1992; **215:** 696–706.
18. Myerson RJ, Michalsi JM, King ML et al, Adjuvant radiation therapy for rectal carcinoma: predictors of outcome. *Int J Radiat Oncol Biol Phys* 1995; **32:** 41–50.
19. Rich TA, Skibber JM, Ajani JA et al, Preoperative infusional chemoradiation for stage T3 rectal cancer. *Int J Radiat Oncol Biol Phys* 1995; **32:** 1025–9.
20. Chan S, Tyler DS, Anscher MS et al, Preoperative radiation and chemotherapy in the treatment of adenocarcinoma of the rectum. *Ann Surg* 1995; **221:** 779–87.
21. Minsky BD, Cohen AM, Kemeny N et al, Enhancement of radiation-induced downstaging of rectal cancer by 5-fluorouracil and high-dose leucovorin chemotherapy. *J Clin Oncol* 1992; **10:** 79–84.
22. Rich TA, Skibber JM, Ajani JA et al, Preoperative infusional chemoradiation therapy for stage T3 rectal cancer. *Int J Radiat Oncol Biol Phys* 1995; **32:** 1025–9.
23. Weinstein GD, Rich TA, Shumate CR et al, Preoperative infusional chemoradiation and surgery with or without an electron beam intraoperative boost for advanced primary rectal cancer. *Int J Radiat Oncol Biol Phys* 1995; **32:** 197–204.
24. Shumate CR, Rich TA, Skibber JM et al, Preoperative chemotherapy and radiation therapy for locally advanced primary and recurrent rectal cancer: a report of surgical morbidity. *Cancer* 1993; **70:** 3690–5.
25. Lowy AM, Rich TA, Skibber JM et al, Preoperative infusional chemoradiation, selective intraoperative radiation and resection for locally advanced pelvic recurrence of colorectal adenocarcinoma. *Ann Surg* 1997; **223:** 177–85.
26. deHaas WG, Miller MJ, Kroll WI et al, Perineal wound closure with the rectus abdominus flap following tumor ablation. *Ann Surg Oncol* 1993; 1: 101–3.
27. Eisenberg B, DeCosse JJ, Harford F, Michalek S, Carcinoma of the colon and rectum: the natural history reviewed in 1704 patients. *Cancer* 1982; **49:** 1131–4.
28. Scheele J, Stangl R, Altendorf-Hofman A, Hepatic metastases from colorectal carcinoma: impact of surgical resection on the natural history. *Br J Surg* 1990; **77:** 1241–6.
29. Adson MA, van Heerden JA, Adson MH et al, Resection of hepatic metastases from colorectal cancer. *Arch Surg* 1984; **119:** 647–51.
30. Hughes K, Simon R, Songhorabodi S et al, Resection of the liver for colorectal carcinoma metastases: a multi-institutional study of indications for resection. *Surgery* 1988; **103:** 278–89.
31. Curley SA, Ehase IL, Roh MS, Hohn DC, Technical considerations and complications associated with the placement of 180 implantable hepatic arterial infusion devices. *Surgery* 1993; **114:** 928–35.
32. Iwatsuki S, Starzl T, Personal experience with 411 hepatic resections. *Ann Surg* 1988; **208:** 421–34.

33. Brown D, Pommier R, Woltering E et al, Nonanatomic hepatic resection for secondary hepatic tumors with special reference to hemostatic technique. *Arch Surg* 1988; **123:** 1063–6.

34. Ravikumar TS, Kane R, Cody B et al, A 5–year study of cryosurgery in the treatment of liver tumors. *Arch Surg* l991; **126:** 1520–4.

35. Ridge J, Bading S, Gelbard A et al, Perfusion of colorectal hepatic metastases: relative distribution of flow from the hepatic artery and portal vein. *Cancer* 1987; **59:** 1547–53.

36. *IMPACT Trial, Efficacy of adjuvant fluorouracil and folinic acid in colon cancer. *Lancet* 1995; **345:** 939–44.

37. O'Connell M, Maillard J, MacDonald J et al, Controlled trial of fluorouracil and low-dose leucovorin given for six months as post-operative adjuvant therapy for colon cancer. *J Clin Oncol* 1997; **15:** 246–50.

38. Wolmark N, Rockette H, Fisher B et al, The benefit of leucovorin modulated 5-fluorouracil as post-operative adjuvant treatment for primary colon cancer: results from the Natl Surg Adjuv Breast and Bowel Project Protocol C-03. *J Clin Oncol* 1993; **11:** 1879–88.

39. *Balzar M, Winter MJ, deBoer CJ, Litvinov SV, The biology of 17-1A antigen (EP-CAM). *J Mol Med* 1999; **77:** 699–712.

40. Gastrointestinal Tumor Study Group, Prolongation of the disease-free survival interval in surgically treated rectal carcinoma. *N Engl J Med* 1985; **312:** 1465–72.

41. Fisher B, Wolmark N, Rockette H et al, Postoperative adjuvant chemotherapy or radiation therapy for rectal cancer: results from NSABP Protocol R-01. *J Natl Cancer Inst* 1988; **80:** 21–9.

42. Krook JE, Moertel CG, Gunderson LL et al, Effective surgical adjuvant therapy for high-risk rectal cancer. *N Engl J Med* 1991; **324:** 709–15.

43. Gastrointestinal Tumor Study Group, Radiation therapy and 5-FU with or without semustine for the treatment of patients with surgical adjuvant adenocarcinoma of the rectum. *J Clin Oncol* 1992; **10:** 549–57.

44. O'Connell MJ, Martenson JA, Wieand HS et al, Improving adjuvant therapy for rectal cancer by combining protracted-infusion 5-FU with radiation therapy after curative surgery. *N Engl J Med* 1994; **331:** 502–7.

45. Willett CG, Haller D, Steele G, Controversies in the management of localized rectal cancer. *ASCO Educational Symposium* 1999: 212–21.

46. *Hoff PM, Lassere Y, Pazdur R, Tegafur and calcium folinate in colorectal cancer: double modulation. *Drugs* 1999; **58**(Suppl 3)**:** 77–83.

47. van Cutsem E, Findlay M, Osterwabler B et al, Capecitabine, an oral fluoropyrimidine carbamate with substantial activity in advanced colorectal cancer. Results of a randomized phase II study. *J Clin Oncol* 2000; **18:** 1337–45.

48. Douilliard JY, Cunningham D, Roth A et al, Irinotecan combined with fluorouracil compared with fluorouracil alone as first-line treatment for metastatic colorectal cancer: a multicenter randomized trial. *Lancet* 2000; **355:** 1041–7.

49. *Levi F, Metzger G, Massari C, Milano G, Oxaliplatin – pharmacokinetics and chronopharmacologic aspects. *Clin Pharmacokinetics* 2000; **38:** 1–21.

50. *Cassileth BR, Complementary and alternative cancer medicine. *J Clin Oncol* 1999; **17:** 44–52.

51. *Berman JM, Chenng RJ, Weinberg DS, Surveillance after colorectal cancer resection. *Lancet* 2000; **355:** 395–9.

The pros and cons of population-based colorectal cancer preventive strategies

Stephen J Spann, Paul Rozen, Bernard Levin, Graeme P Young

Primary prevention: can we prevent colorectal cancer?

The primary prevention of disease is the ultimate goal of any clinician. Is this feasible for colorectal cancer? The answer must logically be yes. Why? Because it is a condition that is occurring with a rapidly rising incidence in countries that have adopted both the negative as well as the positive features of the lifestyle and diet of the westernized world. Preventing these negative aspects from happening and even reversing this trend is the first goal. This is true especially in those areas of Asia, the Mediterranean countries, and Europe where this was not a public health problem until recently (see Chapters 2 and 4).

What about the situation today in countries where habits are so established and seemingly impervious to change, such as the USA, Australia, and South America? The situation is not so immutable. We have examples from the USA where some years ago, cardiovascular disease was occurring in epidemic proportions. Risk factors were identified, including lack of physical activity, overeating saturated fats of meat origin, and not detecting and treating hypertension and hyperlipemia. Within a few years, a concerted public health campaign dramatically reduced the mortality from coronary artery disease. We have also seen the successful results of governmental policy to reduce tobacco smoking, and can look forward to a reduction in tobacco-related diseases.

What about colorectal cancer? As pointed out in Chapter 2, its etiology is multifactorial and seemingly nebulous. There is no single preventable risk factor, but it is the total lifestyle that seems important. This healthy lifestyle is applicable to the prevention of many disorders – cardiovascular, hypertension, diabetes, and some common cancers. A step in this direction has been an overall reduction in meat consumption in Australia and the USA; the success of the Woman's Health Initiative (see Chapter 4) will guide us as to the possibility of changing the long-term lifestyle and dietary habits of large populations.

As pointed out, the maintenance of ideal body weight, reduced consumption of fats, and increased consumption of dietary fiber have salutary effects beyond the primary prevention of colorectal cancer. However, lifestyle modifications do not come easy to individuals, and interventions to promote these have certain costs. Tosteson and colleagues[1] evaluated the cost-effectiveness of promoting a cholesterol-lowering diet at a community level; the marginal cost-effectiveness ratio of lowering the average serum cholesterol by 2% was estimated to be $3200–38 500 per year of life added, but well within the acceptable threshold.

Chemoprevention

What is the place of chemoprevention for colon cancer, as a public health or individual's health policy? Low-dosage aspirin is used to prevent the onset and/or the recurrence of coronary artery disease. Aspirin also reduces some of the risk for colorectal cancer, but there are no recommendations for its use, or for the dosage needed because of the side-effects that occur. This may change with the development of newer and safer medications. In the meantime, we have an armamentarium of naturally occurring and safer products, including olive oil, fish, tea, calcium, and hormone replacement therapy, that experimentally and epidemiologically have been associated with a reduction in colorectal cancer incidence (see Chapter 5).

Secondary prevention: screening for colorectal cancer

What are the potential benefits of screening?

Colorectal cancer is one of the most commonly diagnosed cancers, and a leading cause of cancer deaths, worldwide. The World Health Organization (WHO) estimated that in 1997, there were 875 000 new cases of colon cancer diagnosed, and 510 000 colorectal cancer deaths worldwide.[2] Lieberman[3] has estimated the impact of screening for colorectal cancer in the USA over a 10-year period using various screening methods (Table 10.1). For example, he estimated that a screening program consisting of yearly fecal occult blood testing (FOBT) combined with flexible sigmoidoscopy every 3–5 years, in individuals 50–70 years of age, would prevent 50% of cancers and reduce colorectal cancer mortality by 66%, assuming 100% compliance with the screening program. Thus, if a universal screening program were instituted using these tests, the worldwide incidence of colorectal cancer could potentially be reduced to 437 500 new cases per year, and worldwide mortality reduced to 336 600 deaths per year. The reduction in the number of cancers, and the detection of cancers in earlier stages, would result in a significant reduction in disease and treatment morbidity, as well.

Although early detection through FOBT screening does not seem to lower the costs of eventual colorectal cancer treatment,[4] the reduction in cancer mortality and increase in life expectancy, as well as the ultimate reduction in cancer incidence due to adenomatous polyp detection and removal, will necessarily lead to increased economic productivity in the screened population. From an individual's point of view, early cancer detection and treatment, as well as early polyp identification and removal, should result in increased life expectancy, decreased morbidity, and increased quality of life.

Is population screening feasible?

If we take the example of mammographic screening for breast cancer, this has been implemented successfully worldwide, as a national policy, in many high-risk countries. This required a concerted proactive policy of health authorities and cancer societies. With consistent reinforcement in some countries, population compliance has improved to include the majority of women at risk, with a significant reduction in breast cancer mortality. Its cost has been accepted as feasible for national healthcare, and a similar benefit, but at an even lower cost, has been established for colorectal cancer screening.[5,6]

What are the potential risks of screening for colorectal cancer?

Any healthcare intervention that offers potential benefits also has associated potential risks. The risks associated with screening for colorectal cancer include the risks of false-negative and false-positive tests, the risks of complications of the tests per se, and the risks associated with the treatment of disease identified through the screening process. No screening test is perfectly accurate; any screening test can potentially yield false-negative and false-positive results. False-negative test results are harmful because they offer false reassurance to the screened individual, while resulting in a delay in the diagnosis and treatment of the disease that is being screened for. False-positive test results are harmful because they typically lead to additional diagnostic tests with their costs and own associated risks, or to unnecessary treatment of a supposed disease that isn't really present, with the risks associated with that treatment. Telling an individual that he or she has a positive screening test may result in significant psychological distress, as well.

Table 10.1 *Modeling of impact of screening over a 10-year period on prevention, using various initial screening tools[a]*

Screening test[b]	Compliance (%)	Cancers prevented (%)	Deaths prevented (%)
FOBT alone (annual)	100	22	48
	50	11	24
FS alone (every 3–5 years)	100	38	52
	50	20	30
FS (every 3 years) plus FOBT (annual)	100	50	66
	50	25	33
Barium enema (every 5 years)	100	38	57
	50	19	29
Colonoscopy (every 10 years)	100	70	80
	50	35	40

[a]Adapted from reference 3.
[b]FOBT, fecal occult blood test; FS, flexible sigmoidoscopy.

Consider the case of FOBT screening for colorectal adenomas and cancer. The one-time sensitivity of unrehydrated Hemoccult II slides for the detection of adenomas has been reported to range from 3% to 14% and for the detection of cancer from 18% to 24%.[6] Thus, a patient with adenomatous polyps would have a probability even as high as 97% of having a false-negative test, and being falsely reassured. The specificity of unrehydrated Hemoccult II slides for FOBT has been estimated to be 98%.[6] Thus, a patient without adenoma or colorectal cancer would have a 2% probability of a having a false-positive test. For a 50-year-old American with an average 30% risk of having large-bowel adenomatous polyps, the negative predictive value of a one-time FOBT would be approximately 73%, while the positive predictive value would be around 75%. A negative FOBT alone does not add much reassurance that the patient is free from colorectal adenomas; a positive FOBT substantially increases an individual's probability of having adenomatous polyps. Table 10.2 displays the average sensitivity and specificity of the different screening tests for detecting colorectal adenomas, as well as the positive and negative predictive values of these tests in a 50-year-old at average (30%) risk for such neoplasia.

The most significant risk of flexible sigmoidoscopy, double-contrast barium enema, and colonoscopy is colonic perforation. The risk of perforation from flexible sigmoidoscopy can be as low as 1 in 50 000; the risk from barium enema is around 1 in 10 000. The risk of diagnostic colonoscopy reported after 1980 is about 1 in 2000; the risk of therapeutic colonoscopy reported for the same period was around 1 per 1250 tests. The mortality rate for complications of colonoscopy reported in recent studies is close to 1 per 20 000 examinations, or fewer.[6] These risks must be weighed against the almost 1 in 2 chances of dying from clinically diagnosed colorectal cancer.

What has been patient compliance with colorectal cancer screening recommendations?

Despite the evidence regarding the efficacy of screening tests in reducing colorectal cancer mortality in many communities, at present compliance with screening recommendations is moderate, at best. Vernon[7] performed an extensive literature review of participation in colorectal cancer screening. Rates of patient adherence to FOBT screening varied widely according to the location of the screening program (physician practice, community, or worksite), whether or not the study tested the impact of a specific intervention on screening adherence, and the country in which the study was performed; the median adherence rate among studies was 40–50%. Rescreening rates were found to be less variable, and ranged between 60% and 90%. Rates of patient adherence to sigmoidoscopy were lower, and less variable, as well. Data from the 1992 US National Health Interview Survey showed that only 48% of respondents 49 years and older recalled ever performing an FOBT screen, with only 25% recalling having performed one in the past 3 years, and only 17%

Table 10.2 *The predictive values of various screening tests for colorectal adenomatous polyps in a 50-year-old American at average risk[a]*

Test[b]	Sensitivity (%)	Specificity (%)	Negative predictive value (%)	Positive predictive value (%)
FOBT	14	98	73	75
FS	45	98	81	91
FOBT/FS combination (both tests negative)[c]			83	
DCBE	70	90	88	75
FS/DCBE combination (both tests negative)[c]			93	
Colonoscopy	90	100	96	100

[a]Adapted from reference 6.
[b]FOBT, fecal occult blood test; FS, flexible sigmoidoscopy; DCBE, double-contrast barium enema.
[c]Assumes that 50% of colorectal adenomas will be within the reach of the 60 cm flexible sigmoidoscope.

recalling having performed one within the past year. Only 33% of those respondents recalled ever receiving a sigmoidoscopy examination, with only 9% recalling having received one within the past 3 years, and only 5% recalling having received one within the past year.[8]

In the Minnesota colon cancer control study, the compliance with annual FOBT in the screened group was followed longitudinally.[9] During the first phase of the study (1977–1982), the overall compliance rate was 76.9%; during the second phase (1986–1992), the overall compliance rate was 73.7%. In this study, the guaiac–impregnated paper slides were mailed to screening-group subjects each year; subjects failing to return the cards were sent a reminder letter at 4 weeks, and then telephoned at 10 weeks if these still hadn't been returned. Individuals between the ages of 55 and 80 were more likely to comply with card return, as were women, individuals who lived in the same household with another study participant, and individuals living in metropolitan areas. McCarthy and Moskowitz[10] reported on patient compliance with scheduled screening sigmoidoscopy in an academic general internal medicine practice in Boston. Seventy-five percent of patients scheduled complied with the procedure. Compliance was higher among men and among patients who had family histories of colon cancer.

Lieberman[3] demonstrates the potential impact of compliance on reducing colorectal cancer mortality through a 10-year screening program. He estimates that a program combining annual FOBT with triennial flexible sigmoidoscopy with 100% compliance by the population would reduce colorectal cancer deaths by 66%; with a population compliance of 50%, colorectal cancer mortality would be reduced by 33%; and with a population compliance of 25%, the colorectal cancer mortality would be reduced by only 21%.

How can compliance with colorectal cancer screening recommendations be increased?

Cancer screening programs can be implemented at a community (or population) level, and at a physician practice (or individual patient) level. A number of lessons have been learned from breast cancer screening programs, which are probably generalizable to screening for colorectal cancer. Individual participant (or patient) compliance can be enhanced through a number of interventions. Improved knowledge about the disease and the benefits of screening improves compliance. The public can be educated about the importance of screening through the use of mass communications media, such as newspapers, television, and billboards. Well-known personalities such as politicians, actors, etc. who have experienced the disease can be powerful advocates for screening, as can immediate family members. The receipt of written educational materials and a written or telephone invitation or reminder to participate in a screening intervention can increase individual compliance.[11] Involving the patient in the decision to be screened improves patient compliance with cancer screening interventions.[12]

Physician and practice compliance with screening programs can also be improved through a number of interventions. The existence of a specific screening guideline motivates physicians to carry out screening interventions. Improved knowledge by physicians of the efficacy and effectiveness of the screening intervention enhances physician compliance, as well.[13] This can be achieved through continuing medical education programs and academic detailing. The costs for any test have to be adequate to compensate for physician effort. If not, then there is little incentive to promote screening. The German National FOBT Screening Program has exemplified this, where there had been poor physician compliance until recent improvement in physician compensation (Dr R Gnauck, personal communication). Coverage of the intervention by third-party insurers is also a positive incentive.[14]

Systems to help remind the physician when specific preventive interventions are due help improve compliance with screening. A health maintenance flow sheet, which shows when specific interventions are due and allows a place to record their completion, is useful (Figure 10.1). Colored stickers placed on the patient's chart can serve as a reminder to obtain certain screening tests at certain intervals.[15] Physician reminders about preventive interventions due can be generated by computer at each visit to enhance compliance with screening guidelines.[16] Either a computerized billing system or a computerized medical record system can be programmed to accomplish this task. Patient-recall systems are also helpful for reminding patients when it is time for specific screening tests. These can be as simple as a card-based reminder file system, or as sophisticated as a computerized system based on a practice billing system or computerized medical record. A card-based reminder file can be developed by completing a reminder postcard with the patient's mailing address, which is then placed in a box that has dividers organized according to future dates. If Mr Smith is on a once-yearly FOBT screening protocol and completes the test in June 2000, then a reminder postcard is completed and placed in the reminder file box behind the divider for June 2001. On June 1, 2001, all cards behind that divider will be removed and mailed, and Mr Smith will receive his reminder that he is due for his yearly FOBT. Practices can develop continuous quality-improvement programs,

Preventive intervention	Age																									
	50	51	52	53	54	55	56	57	58	59	60	61	62	63	64	65	66	67	68	69	70	71	72	73	74	75
Weight	*	*	*	*	*	*	*	*	*	*	*	*	*	*	*	*	*	*	*	*	*	*	*	*	*	*
Blood pressure	*	*	*	*	*	*	*	*	*	*	*	*	*	*	*	*	*	*	*	*	*	*	*	*	*	*
Tetanus–diphtheria booster	*										*										*					
Influenza vaccine	*	*	*	*	*	*	*	*	*	*	*	*	*	*	*	*	*	*	*	*	*	*	*	*	*	*
Pneumococcal vaccine																*										
Pap smear	*			*			*			*			*			*			*			*			*	
Clinical breast examination	*	*	*	*	*	*	*	*	*	*	*	*	*	*	*	*	*	*	*	*	*	*	*	*	*	*
Mammograms	*	*	*	*	*	*	*	*	*	*	*	*	*	*	*	*	*	*	*	*	*	*	*	*	*	*
FOBT	*	*	*	*	*	*	*	*	*	*	*	*	*	*	*	*	*	*	*	*	*	*	*	*	*	*
Flexible sigmoidoscopy	*					*					*					*					*					*
Discuss DRE and PSA	*	*	*	*	*	*		*	*	*	*	*	*	*	*	*	*	*	*	*	*	*	*	*	*	*
Serum cholesterol	*					*					*					*					*					*

Figure 10.1 *Flowchart of preventive medical examinations that a family physician needs to perform. FOBT, fecal occult blood test; DRE, digital rectal examination; PSA, prostate-specific antigen.*

involving recursive measurements of physician compliance with specific prevention guidelines. Practices involved with such programs typically strive to show continuous improvement in their performance. The use of physician practice pattern audits against certain external quality markers, developed and carried out by certain external agencies, also serve as an incentive to enhance physician compliance with screening interventions. One example is the Health Plan Employer Data and Information Set (HEDIS) criteria established by the National Committee on Quality Assurance (NCQA);[17] these are used by US managed care organizations seeking NCQA accreditation, in the audit of provider physician practices. Current HEDIS criteria include screening for breast and cervical cancer.

Involving non-physician office personnel in managing a screening program through protocols has also been shown to increase compliance with cancer screening.[18] To some extent, these preventive measures can be delegated to nurse–practitioners, but the physician has a crucial role in initiating discussion of the topic, including a warm recommendation to follow through with implementation. In some medical systems, there is centralized managed preventive care for promoting and organizing mammographic screening. If there is, it would seem more cost-efficient to add colorectal cancer screening to this framework. In summary, there are a number of methods, that can be utilized to enhance compliance with cancer screening recommendations; these are summarized in Table 10.3.

What are patient attitudes and preferences for colorectal cancer screening tests?

Several studies have evaluated patient attitudes and preferences for the different colorectal cancer screening tests. Leard and colleagues[19] asked 100 patients aged 50–75 years from three primary-care practices in San Diego, California which of five different colorectal cancer screening options they would choose, how likely they would be to undergo each of the options, and whether or not they would undergo the test if recommended. Colonoscopy was the screening test that most (38%) selected as their first choice. FOBT was the test that most ranked as highly likely that they would undergo, and that most would undergo if the test was recommended. Patients who had previously undergone colonoscopy were most likely to choose this test as their preferred screening option (Table 10.4).

Pignone and colleagues[20] evaluated patient preferences for four different colorectal cancer screening strategies in 146 adults in an adult university internal medicine practice in North Carolina. Patient preferences were measured at three points: after descriptive information about colon cancer and screening options; after information about test performance but with no out-of-pocket costs; and finally with hypothetical out-of-pocket costs. After receiving descriptive information about testing procedures, most (45%) chose the FOBT-alone option. Following receipt of information on test performance, most preferred the FOBT plus flexible sigmoidoscopy option. After receiving the out-of-pocket cost information, most preferred the FOBT alone strategy (Table 10.5). Dominitz and Provenzale[21] used the time trade-off method to measure patient preferences for flexible sigmoidoscopy and colonoscopy, each to be performed every 5 years for 20 years. Four different groups of patients aged 50–75 years were identified at the Veterans Administration Hospital in Durham, North Carolina: unscreened patients who had

Table 10.3 *Methods to enhance compliance with cancer screening*

Target	Method
Individual participant (patient)	• Improve knowledge through public education • Provide written educational materials, written and/or telephone invitation/reminder to participate • Involve the patient in the decision to screen
Physician/ practice	• Provide specific screening guidelines • Cover cost of intervention through health insurance • Educate the physician about the efficacy and effectiveness of screening • Reminder systems: health maintenance flow sheets, chart stickers, computer-generated reminders • Patient-recall systems: card-based reminder file, computer-generated • Continuous quality-improvement program • External audits • Involve non-physician office personnel through protocols

Table 10.4 *Patient preferences of test options as assessed by three different approaches[a]*

	No screening	Fecal occult blood test (FOBT)	Flexible sigmoidoscopy	Barium enema	Colonoscopy
Percentage of patients who selected test as first preference[b]	4	31	13	14	38
Mean likelihood of patients undergoing test (1 = highly unlikely, 5 = highly likely)[c]	1.6	4.4	3.4	3.4	3.4
Percentage of patients who would undergo test if recommended[d]	—	96	82	92	86
Percentage of patients who have had this test and who prefer this screening test[e]	14	36	17	15	71

[a]Adapted from reference 19.
[b]Colonoscopy versus FOBT, $p = 0.40$; colonoscopy versus barium enema, $p = 0.0007$; FOBT versus barium enema, $p = 0.01$.
[c]FOBT versus colonoscopy, $p < 0.0001$.
[d]FOBT versus colonoscopy, $p = 0.01$.
[e]Colonoscopy versus FOBT, $p < 0.0001$.

never undergone colorectal cancer screening; screened patients who were undergoing flexible sigmoidoscopy; 'cooperative study' patients who were enrolled in a multicenter prospective study of risk factors for large adenomas of the colon and were about to undergo colonoscopy; and colorectal cancer patients who had previously been diagnosed with and treated for colorectal cancer. Unscreened patients were willing to give up significantly more time (life expectancy) to avoid screening sigmoidoscopy and colonoscopy (median 91 days and 183 days, respectively) than were patients undergoing screening sigmoidoscopy (median 0 days and 7 days, respectively) or screening colonoscopy (median 0 days and 0 days, respectively), or patients with colorectal cancer (median 0

Table 10.5 *Subjects' preferences for colon cancer screening (n = 146)[a]*

Specific strategy[b]	Descriptive information on testing procedure (%)	Test performance information, no out-of-pocket costs (%)	Test performance information, with out-of-pocket costs (%)
FOBT alone	45	36	53
FS alone	13	12	8
FOBT and FS	38	47[c]	31[d]
Colonoscopy	1	1	2
Neither	3	3	5
Unable to answer	1	1	1

[a]Reprinted by permission of Blackwell Science, Inc., from the *Journal of General Internal Medicine*, 1999; **14:** 434.
[b]FOBT, fecal occult blood test; FS, flexible sigmoidoscopy.
[c]$p = 0.12$; [d]$p < 0.001$.

days and 0 days, respectively). These studies suggest that patients are most likely to choose, and comply with, FOBT screening over more invasive screening procedures. On the other hand, patients who have already decided to undergo, or have previously experienced, invasive tests are much less reluctant to have these performed.

Patients often find that invasive screening procedures are not as embarrassing, uncomfortable, or painful as they had feared they would be. McCarthy and Moskowitz[10] found that 41.1% of individuals undergoing screening flexible sigmoidoscopy expected to experience moderate to extreme embarrassment, but only 27.4% actually did; 55.5% expected to experience moderate to extreme discomfort, but only 41.7% did; and 40.8% expected to experience moderate to extreme pain, but only 30.9% did. When asked about their willingness to have screening sigmoidoscopy again, 25.7% said they probably would, and 63.5% said they definitely would. Cockburn and colleagues[22] evaluated the acceptance of screening flexible sigmoidoscopy in 187 general-practice patients, aged 50 – 60 years, in Melbourne, Australia. Forty-nine percent of patients received the recommended sigmoidoscopy: 65% experienced either no or mild discomfort; while 15% experienced moderate or severe pain. Eighty percent experienced a bloated feeling, but only 36% felt moderate or extreme bloating. Sixty-four percent experienced no embarrassment, though 9% reported moderate to extreme embarrassment.

It has been shown that recommendation by the family or treating physician is crucial in initiating a particular screening test. This has been demonstrated successfully in the UK and Norway, where there have been an overall 40% agreement to participate and a 70% compliance for a sigmoidoscopy screening program that included tens of thousands of persons in defined geographic areas of both countries (Dr W Atkin and Dr G Hoff, personal communications). However, in other countries, national prejudices in the average-risk population would inhibit cooperation with such an invasive screening procedure (personal communication, Dr M Crespi, Rome).

What are the economics of screening for colorectal cancer?

In every country, healthcare resources are limited, while healthcare needs are limitless. Rationing decisions about allocation of healthcare resources are inevitable. With advances in modern medical technology, there are a growing number of healthcare interventions that have been proven to be efficacious and effective. The problem is that no society can afford to implement all of them. Some interventions are cost-saving: they save more in downstream healthcare expenditures than they cost. Most interventions, however, are not cost-saving: their implementation would add incremental healthcare costs to society, while yielding incremental (improvement in) health. Since policymakers are frequently forced to choose among several potentially effective healthcare interventions for implementation, they need a methodology to help them make rationing decisions. Cost-effectiveness analysis is a methodology that allows policymakers to compare healthcare interventions by evaluating the relative cost per unit of outcome achieved by a given intervention. Costs are typically expressed in monetary units: dollars, pounds, francs, etc. Outcomes may be expressed in a number of ways: cancers diagnosed, deaths prevented, years of life saved, etc. Since a year of life with cancer is not equal to a year of life with heart disease, life-expectancy outcomes are typically normalized (quality-adjusted) to a state of perfect health, and expressed as quality-adjusted life-years (QALYs). Individuals value different health states according to their personal preferences or 'utilities'; utilities are typically expressed as a value between 1 (perfect health) and 0 (death). Quality-adjusted life expectancy (in QALYs) is obtained by multiplying the life expectancy in a given health state by the individual's utility for that health state.[23] Thus, if an individual has been diagnosed with Dukes C stage colon cancer and has a life expectancy of 5 years, and a utility of 0.95 for his post-treatment health state, then his quality-adjusted life expectancy is 4.75 QALYs. A cost-effectiveness analysis that expresses outcomes in terms of quality-adjusted life expectancy is called a 'cost-utility' analysis. A marginal cost-effectiveness (or cost-utility) analysis compares the relative costs and outcomes of two interventions:[23]

$$\text{marginal cost-effectiveness ratio} = \frac{(C_2 - C_1)}{(E_2 - E_1)}$$

where C_2 is the cost of intervention 2, C_1 is the cost of intervention 1, E_2 is the effectiveness of intervention 2, and E_1 is the effectiveness of intervention 1.

Marginal cost-effectiveness analyses can be utilized to compare various intervention strategies designed to achieve the same outcome; for example, as we shall see below, Wagner and colleagues[6] have performed an analysis comparing the marginal cost-effectiveness of various strategies for screening for colorectal cancer. This type of analysis may also be used to decide whether the cost-effectiveness of a given intervention is comparable to that of other healthcare interventions that have already been accepted and implemented. This requires a 'threshold' range of acceptability. In the USA, for example, a health-care intervention is currently considered to be cost-effective if its marginal cost-effectiveness ratio is under $50 000 per QALY saved.[24]

Cost-effectiveness analysis typically involves the development of a statistical model, or decision tree, which seeks to represent the various interventions that are being considered, along with the various potential outcomes for each intervention, and the probability of each one of those outcomes. The cost and the health outcomes are then estimated for each intervention. Cost-effectiveness analysis modeling is a complicated exercise, and must take into account all of the variables that affect the outcomes of the intervention.[23]

A number of studies have been published that evaluate the cost-effectiveness of various testing strategies screen-

ing for colorectal cancer. Wagner and colleagues[6] constructed a model to evaluate the potential health outcomes and costs of 16 different colorectal cancer screening strategies over the remaining lifetimes of a cohort of 50-year-old individuals. The following screening strategies were modeled:

- annual FOBT;
- flexible sigmoidoscopy every 3, 5, or 10 years;
- double-contrast barium enema every 3, 5, or 10 years;
- colonoscopy every 3, 5, or 10 years;
- annual FOBT and flexible sigmoidoscopy every 3, 5, or 10 years;
- annual FOBT and double-contrast barium enema every 3, 5, or 10 years.

The variables and base-case value assumptions used in this model are listed in Table 10.6.[6] The marginal cost-effectiveness ratio of each screening strategy (compared with no screening) estimated by the model using the base-case assumptions and a 10-year polyp dwell time are shown in Table 10.7. The marginal cost-effectiveness ratios range from $9406 for annual FOBT, to $10 541 per year of life added for flexible sigmoidoscopy every 5 years, to $11 652 if annual FOBT is added, to $12 750 per year of life added for colonoscopy every 5 years (Figure 10.2). In the USA, only by reducing the costs of endoscopic procedures would periodic endoscopy be cost-effective and comparable to FOBT as a screening method.

Patient utilities for the different health outcome states were not included in this analysis. However, Whynes and colleagues[25] took patients diagnosed with colorectal cancer in the Nottingham FOBT screening trial to evaluate their quality of life following surgery for colorectal cancer, and to compare the quality of life between patients whose cancer was detected by screening with that of patients whose cancer presented symptomatically. The mode of entry to diagnosis and treatment (screening versus no screening) did not appear to affect post-intervention quality-of-life. The stage of cancer progression was not closely related to outcome quality of life, either. A quality-of-life adjustment coefficient for surviving patients was estimated to lie within the range of 0.95–0.98. When the life-expectancy outcomes in the Wagner model are quality-adjusted utilizing a coefficient of 0.95, the marginal cost-utility ratios still fall well within the range of what is typically considered to be cost-effective.

In an older model Eddy,[26] using different data, also evaluated the cost-effectiveness of a number of different

Table 10.6 *Cost-effectiveness analysis of colorectal cancer screening strategies: summary of assumptions*[a]

Parameter[b]	Base-case value[c]
Sensitivity/specificity of screening and diagnosis	
Sensitivity of FOBT for polyps	10%
Sensitivity of FOBT for cancer	60%
Sensitivity of colonoscopy for polyps/cancer	90%
Sensitivity of DCBE for polyps/cancer	70%
Sensitivity of FS for polyps/cancer	90%
Reach of FS	50%
Specificity of FOBT	90%
Specificity of colonoscopy	100%
Specificity of FS	98%
Specificity of DCBE	90%
Natural history of polyp/cancer sequence	
Prevalence of polyps at age 50 years	30%
Annual polyp incidence rate	Age-specific: 50–65 years: 1.33% per year; 66–70 years: 2% per year; >70 years: 1% per year
Percentage of cancers originating as polyps	70%
Annual cancer incidence with no screening	Age-specific, based on SEER data
Percentage of cancers detected in early stage with no screening	40%
Dwelling time of cancer in early stage	2 years
Percentage of total dwelling time in early stage before clinical detection (0–100%)	100%
Dwelling time of cancer in late stage before detection	2 years
Five-year all-cause survival for early cancer	Age-specific, based on SEER data
5-year all-cause survival for late cancer	Age-specific, based on SEER data
Precancerous polyp dwelling time detectable by FS, DCBE, colonoscopy	10 years
Precancerous polyp dwelling time detectable by FOBT	10 years
Complications and unintended consequences	
Rate of perforation of colon in colonoscopy	0.0007
Death rate from colonoscopy	0.00005
Rate of colonic perforation from DCBE, FS	0.0
Surgical mortality rate from colonic resection	2%
Prevalence of lifetime-latent cancers at age 50 years	0.2%
Annual incidence of lifetime-latent cancers	Age-specific: 50–65 years: 0.02%; 65–85 years: 0.05%
Costs	
Unit cost of screening FOBT	$10
Unit cost of screening FS	$80
Unit cost of screening DCBE	$131
Unit cost of screening colonoscopy	$285
Unit cost of diagnostic colonoscopy	$285
Unit cost of diagnostic colonoscopy with polypectomy	$434
Unit cost of surveillance colonoscopy	$285
Unit cost of tissue pathology for polyps and lesions	$64
Lifetime cost of treating early cancer	$35 000
Lifetime cost of treating late cancer	$45 000
Lifetime cost of treating perforated colon	$35 000
Discount rate	5% per year

[a]Adapted from reference 6.
[b]DCBE, double-contrast barium enema; FOBT, fecal occult blood test; FS, flexible sigmoidoscopy.
[c]SEER, Surveillance, Epidemiology and End Results tumor registry system funded by the US National Cancer Institute, Bethesda, Maryland.

Table 10.7 Cost-effectiveness of colorectal cancer: base-case assumptions and 10-year polyp dwell time[a]

Strategy[b]	Years of life gained per 100 000 persons screened (000s)	Added cost per 100 000 persons screened ($ millions)	Cost per added year of life ($)
Annual FOBT	5.88	58.2	9906
FS every 3 years	3.99	51.9	13001
FS every 5 years	3.58	37.8	10541
FS every 10 years	3.13	24.9	7966
FS every 3 years and annual FOBT	6.78	89.3	13180
FS every 5 years and annual FOBT	6.72	78.3	11652
FS every 10 years and annual FOBT	6.64	70.0	10526
DCBE every 3 years	6.72	74.7	11115
DCBE every 5 years	6.02	56.8	9435
DCBE every 10 years	4.78	44.1	9224
DCBE every 3 years and annual FOBT	7.47	112.1	14996
DCBE every 5 years and annual FOBT	7.33	93.9	12815
DCBE every 10 years and annual FOBT	7.06	80.7	11444
Colonoscopy every 3 years	6.82	118.8	17424
Colonoscopy every 5 years	6.5	82.9	12750
Colonoscopy every 10 years	5.93	55.1	9287

[a]Adapted from reference 6.
[b]DCBE, double-contrast barium enema; FOBT, fecal occult blood test; FS, flexible sigmoidoscopy.

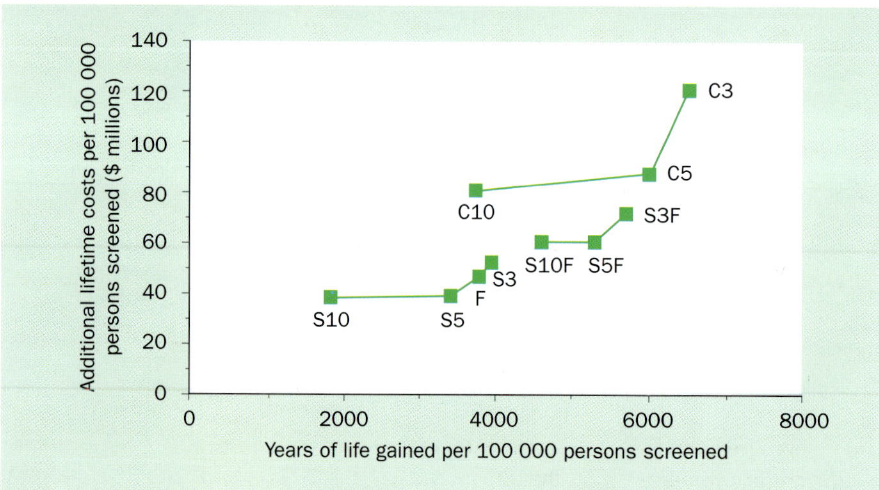

Figure 10.2 Years of life gained versus costs for three commonly performed screening strategies at age 50 years: annual fecal occult blood test (FOBT) alone (F); annual FOBT and periodic flexible sigmoidoscopy (S) at 3-, 5-, or 10-year intervals; colonoscopy (C), at 3-, 5-, or 10-year intervals. Adapted from reference 6, Figure 19.2a.

strategies for screening for colorectal cancer. For a 50-year-old male, he estimated the following marginal cost-effectiveness ratios: annual FOBT, $8378 per added year of life; annual FOBT plus double-contrast barium enema every 5 years, $12202 per year of life added; and annual FOBT plus flexible sigmoidoscopy every 5 years, $19196 per year of life added. Whynes and colleagues[27] developed a cost-utility analysis model using data from the Nottingham FOBT screening trial. For individuals initiating biennial FOBT screening at age 50 and continuing to age 74 years, the estimated marginal cost-utility is £2127 per QALY gained for males, and £1426 per QALY gained for females. Gyrd-Hansen and colleagues[28] utilized data from the Funen screening trial in Denmark to evaluate the cost-effectiveness of colorectal cancer screening using FOBT, modeling a number of different screening intervals, as well as age groups targeted for the program. Marginal cost-effectiveness ratios ranged from DKr 17 000 per life-year added for screening individuals 65–74 years of age biennially to DKr 42 500 per life-year added for screening individuals 50–74 years of age every year (DKr 1 = $ 0.15).

Loeve et al.[29] developed a model to evaluate the cost-effectiveness of colorectal cancer screening using every 5-year sigmoidoscopy over a 30-year period. This model estimated a cost savings of $5 per person screened: the costs of screening, diagnosis, polypectomy, and ongoing surveillance of individuals found to have polyps was $5 less than the costs of treatment, continuous care, and terminal care in individuals diagnosed at the onset of symptoms. This model estimated that there would also be 28 years of life gained per 1000 individuals in the screening program.

How does the cost-effectiveness of colorectal cancer screening compare with that of screening for other cancers? Lindfors and Rosenquist[5] evaluated breast cancer screening using effectiveness estimates derived from a variety of sources, including trials conducted in the UK, Sweden, and the USA. The marginal cost-effectiveness ratios varied, depending on the frequency of screening and the age group screened. For women aged 50–79 years, the ratio for annual mammography was estimated at $31 000 per year of life added; this fell to $19 000 per year of life added for biennial screening programs. Eddy[30] estimated that the marginal cost-effectiveness ratio for cervical cancer screening with every-4-year Pap smears in women aged 20–75 years was $14 000 per year of life added. The cost-effectiveness of colorectal cancer screening compares favorably with both that of breast cancer and that of cervical cancer screening.

The cost-effectiveness of other preventive interventions has also been estimated. Edelson and colleagues[31] estimated the marginal cost-effectiveness ratio for treating hypertension with hydrochlorothiazide to be $16 400 per year of life added. Goldman and colleagues[32] estimated the cost-effectiveness of primary prevention of coronary artery disease by treating individuals with hypercholesterolemia using lovastatin; the cost-effectiveness ratios varied according to individual risk status. For males aged 45–54 years who were smokers, moderately hypertensive, 130% or more of ideal body weight, with a serum cholesterol level of 300 mg/dl (7.76 mmol/l) or more, the cost-effectiveness ratio was estimated to be $22 000 per year of life added. The cost-effectiveness of colorectal cancer screening compares favorably with those of all of these preventive interventions.

Colorectal cancer screening and national health policy

Given that colorectal cancer screening has been shown to be efficacious, acceptable to individuals, and cost-effective, one would anticipate that routine periodic screening for this disease would be common health policy in most countries. This, in fact, is not the case – but it is changing. The WHO recommends yearly FOBT and digital rectal examination and flexible sigmoidoscopy every 3–5 years in all asymptomatic individuals, beginning at age 50 years.[33] In the USA, in 1995, the Preventive Services Task Force[34] recommended periodic screening for colorectal cancer in individuals 50–75 years of age. Medicare, the national health insurance plan for the elderly, began to pay for periodic screening tests for colorectal cancer, effective January 1, 1998. Screening FOBT is covered at a frequency of every 12 months, and screening flexible sigmoidoscopy is covered at a frequency of once every 48 months, for individuals 50 years old and above who have Medicare insurance. Screening colonoscopy is covered at a frequency of once every 24 months for individuals at high risk for colorectal cancer (positive family history, prior colorectal cancer or precursor neoplastic polyps, history of inflammatory bowel disease, the presence of any appropriate gene markers for colorectal cancer, or other predisposing factors). Since July 2001, Medicare covers screening colonoscopy at a frequency of every 10 years for individuals at average risk of colorectal cancer. Screening barium enema may be substituted for either a screening flexible sigmoidoscopy or a screening colonoscopy.[35] This screening policy for average- and high-risk groups has been adopted by many of the US medical insurance companies (Table 10.8).

In Japan, a yearly 2-day immunochemical FOBT screen is offered to individuals over the age of 40 years.[36] While the European Group for Colorectal Cancer Screening strongly recommends the implementation of repeated FOBT screening for asymptomatic individuals 50 years of age and older,[37] health policy on this issue varies by country within Europe. While Germany, the Czech Republic, and Israel promote FOBT colorectal cancer screening in asymptomatic individuals beginning at age 50 years, the UK has yet to implement such a recommendation as a national policy.[38,39] However, pilot fecal occult blood studies are planned for defined geographical areas in the UK, and a large-scale flexible sigmoidoscopy and polypectomy program has completed enrollment and the investigators are awaiting follow-up results on cancer incidence and

Table 10.8 *Colorectal cancer screening guidelines for individuals at average risk: major US health maintenance organizations (HMOs)*

HMO	Guidelines (age ≥ 50 years)
Aetna/U.S. Healthcare	Fecal occult blood test, annually, and/or sigmoidoscopy
Cigna Health Care	Fecal occult blood test, annually; sigmoidoscopy, at clinical discretion
Humana	Fecal occult blood test, annually, and/or sigmoidoscopy every 3–5 years
Kaiser Permanente	Fecal occult blood test annually, or flexible sigmoidoscopy every 10 years
PacifiCare	Fecal occult blood test, annually; flexible sigmoidoscopy every 48 months; barium enema examinations as alternative to sigmoidoscopy

mortality. Norway does not yet recommend population colorectal cancer screening, despite a cost-effectiveness analysis of a one-time sigmoidoscopy examination at age 60 years, modeled on Norwegian data, which showed a favorable marginal cost-effectiveness ratio.[40] However, the original study has been extended to defined geographical areas, and the populations at risk are offered flexible sigmoidoscopy and an immunochemcial FOBT (FlexSure) that has a high specificity and will not lead to an excessive number of colonoscopic examinations.[38] In Italy, a 5-yearly screening colonoscopic examination is now being offered to the average-risk population (personal communication, Dr M Crespi, Rome). In Australia, the Health Technology Advisory Committee of the National Health and Medical Research Council recently concluded that screening for colorectal cancer in that country shows sufficient promise to warrant exploration through the establishment of pilot and feasibility studies and recommending the introduction of population screening by FOBT for the average-risk population over age 50 years.[41] Four nationally budgeted pilot FOBT studies are now being initiated in defined geographical areas.

In New Zealand, the National Advisory Committee on Health and the Disability Working Party on Population Screening for Colorectal Cancer recently recommended against population-based screening for colorectal cancer because of the costs.[42] They do perform breast cancer screening. The Canadian Task Force on the Periodic Health Examination also does not recommend periodic colorectal cancer screening.[43]

Why do such discrepancies exist in colorectal cancer screening policies between developed countries? Although cost-effective compared to other healthcare interventions, colorectal cancer screening may not be viewed as affordable by health policymakers in some countries. Initiation of such a program will generate an increase in healthcare costs. Whynes[44] has estimated that the incremental cost to the UK National Health Service for implementing a biennial FOBT screening program in individuals aged 45–74 years would be £40 million per year. This figure does not include the extra costs of treatment, and the investment necessary to establish the national screening infrastructure, including the provision of additional capacity for evaluating positive FOBTs, manpower training, and the development of call–recall systems for the invitation of subjects. The addition of such a screening program would require either an overall increase in healthcare expenditures, which some countries are not prepared to incur, or the shifting of resources away from some other, established, healthcare intervention to the new screening program: in a system with finite resources, there is an opportunity cost to implementing a new program, which means the loss of opportunity to continue some other, established, intervention.[39] Some countries are awaiting the results of randomized clinical trials testing other methods of colorectal cancer screening,[44] or the results of pilot programs implemented within the country on a trial basis.[41]

How will the family physician manage?

The primary-care giver is subject to numerous competing demands. Not only does he or she have to manage the medical problem that brought the patient to their attention, but they are expected to provide a battery of preventive health recommendations for the patient: examine for hypertension, hyperlipidemia, and mammography, deal with tobacco smoking and obesity, and now add colorectal cancer screening.

While cost-effectiveness analysis data may be useful to healthcare policymakers trying to decide how to allocate healthcare resources, they may be less useful to the physician faced with trying to implement several preventive interventions with his or her patients, and to the patient, who has to decide with which of those interventions he or she will choose to comply. If the patient's health insurance covers the proposed preventive interventions, then the 'scarce' resources that necessitate prioritization are the physician's time and energy, and the patient's willingness to undergo the screening intervention, or (in the case of primary prevention) to change health habits and lifestyle. How are the physician and the patient to prioritize among potential preventive interventions? One option is to prioritize based on the effectiveness of the potential interventions. Wright and Weinstein[45] have compiled effectiveness data, in terms of average gains in life expectancy, for several medical interventions, based on a number of decision and cost-effectiveness analyses. Table 10.9 summarizes some of the findings of their study, and may be useful to physicians and patients in prioritizing among potential preventive interventions. The incremental life-expectancy estimates reflect the *average* increase in life expectancy gained by every individual participating in the specific intervention. An individual who develops a cancer and is diagnosed at an early asymptomatic stage will benefit by an increase in life expectancy that is much greater than the estimated average, while an individual who never develops a cancer will receive no benefit from the screening in terms of increased life expectancy.

Are there legal obligations to promote colorectal cancer screening?

There are now precedents where the treating physician has been successfully sued for negligence for not recommending preventive medical examinations to family members at risk and having a defined inherited risk for cancer (see Chapter 6). At present, there are various national recommendations or screening guidelines for the average-risk population. What are the medicolegal implications of national (or international) policies or guidelines for colorectal cancer screening? What liability does a physician assume if he or she doesn't recommend FOBT screening on an annual basis, and flexible sigmoidoscopy screening on an every-5-year basis to a 55-year-old patient at average risk, who is later diagnosed with an advanced-stage colorectal carcinoma, in a country with a national colorectal cancer screening policy? Will the courts consider this an act of medical negligence by omission? While there is no substantial case law on this subject at this time, we can only speculate that this could eventually become an important cause for litigation. While physicians should base their practice on the best available evidence and doing what is best for their patients, the specter of malpractice litigation can be a powerful

Table 10.9 *Effectiveness of various preventive interventions by gain in life expectancy*[a]

Disease/intervention	Target population	Average gain in life expectancy (months)	
		Males	**Females**
Breast cancer/ 10 years of biennial mammograms	50-year-old women	—	0.8
Cervical cancer/ Pap smear every 3 years for 55 years[30]	20-year-old women	—	3.1
Colon cancer/ Annual fecal occult blood test and flexible sigmoidoscopy every 5 years for 25 years[26]	50-year-olds	1.6	1.5
Reduction of diastolic blood pressure to 88 mmHg	35-year-olds with hypertension, diastolic blood pressure 90–94 mmHg	13	11
Reduction of cholesterol to 200 mg/dl (5.2 mmol/l)	35-year-olds with hypercholesterolemia of 200–239 mg/dl (5.2–6.2 mmol/l)	6	5

[a]Adapted from reference 45.

force in shaping physician behavior. It would seem prudent for the treating physician to offer the screening standard of care accepted in that particular community or medical insurance group.

Conclusions

In conclusion, a strong case can be made for the primary and secondary prevention of colorectal cancer. The potential benefits of prevention significantly outweigh the potential risks. Colorectal cancer screening has been shown to be of comparable cost-effectiveness to other common preventive healthcare interventions. There are significant medicolegal reasons why physicians should encourage their patients to participate in colorectal cancer screening programs. And there are a number of proven methods for increasing both physician/practice compliance and patient compliance with screening recommendations.

References (*Reviews and general articles)

1. Tosteson AN, Weinstein MC, Hunink MG et al, Cost-effectiveness of populationwide educational approaches to reduce serum cholesterol levels. *Circulation* 1997; **95:** 24–30.

2. *World Health Organization, *The World Health Report*. Geneva: WHO, 1997.

3. *Lieberman D, Mass screening: North American perspective. In: *Prevention and Early Detection of Colorectal Cancer* (Young GP, Rozen P, Levin B, eds). London: Saunders, 1996: 289–300.

4. Whynes DK, Walker AR, Chamberlain JO et al, Screening and the costs of treating colorectal cancer. *Br J Cancer* 1993; **68:** 965–8.

5. Lindfors KK, Rosenquist CJ, The cost-effectiveness of mammographic screening strategies. *JAMA* 1995; **274:** 881–4.

6. *Wagner JL, Tunis S, Brown M et al, Cost-effectiveness of colorectal cancer screening in average-risk adults. In: *Prevention and Early Detection of Colorectal Cancer* (Young GP, Rozen P, Levin B, eds). London: Saunders, 1996: 321–41.

7. *Vernon SW, Participation in colorectal cancer screening: a review, *J Natl Cancer Inst* 1997; **89:** 1406–21.

8. Anderson LM, May DS, Has the use of cervical, breast, and colorectal cancer screening increased in the United States? *Am J Public Health* 1995; **85:** 840–2.

9. Thomas W, White CM, Mah J et al, Longitudinal compliance with annual screening for fecal occult blood. *Am J Epidemiol* 1995; **142:** 176–82.

10. McCarthy BD, Moskowitz MA, Screening flexible sigmoidoscopy: patient attitudes and compliance. *J Gen Intern Med* 1993; **8:** 120–5.

11. Saywell RM Jr, Champion VL, Skinner CS et al, Cost-effectiveness comparison of five interventions to increase mammography screening. *Prev Med* 1999; **29:** 374–82.

12. Phillips KA, Kerlikowske K, Baker LC et al, Factors associated with women's adherence to mammography screening guidelines. *Health Serv Res* 1998; **33:** 29–53.

13. Costanza ME, Stoddard AM, Zapka JG et al, Physician compliance with mammography guidelines: barriers and enhancers. *J Am Board Fam Pract* 1992; **5:** 143–52.

14. May DS, Kiefe CI, Funkhouser E et al, Compliance with mammography guidelines: physician recommendation and patient adherence. *Prev Med* 1999; **28:** 386–94.

15. Grady KE, Lemkau JP, Lee NR et al, Enhancing mammography referral in primary care. *Prev Med* 1997; **26:** 791–800.

16. Yarnall KS, Rimer BK, Hynes D et al, Computerized prompts for cancer screening in a community health center. *J Am Board Fam Pract* 1998; **11:** 96–104.

17. http://www.ncqa.org/pages/policy/hedis/h00meas.htm.

18. McCarthy BD, Yood MU, Bolton MB et al, Redesigning primary care processes to improve the offering of mammography. The use of clinic protocols by nonphysicians. *J Gen Intern Med* 1997; **12:** 357–63.

19. Leard LE, Savides TJ, Ganiats TG, Patient preferences for colorectal cancer screening. *J Fam Pract* 1997; **45:** 211–8.

20. Pignone M, Bucholtz D, Harris R, Patient preferences for colon cancer screening. *J Gen Intern Med* 1999; **14:** 432–7.

21. Dominitz JA, Provenzale D, Patient preferences and quality of life associated with colorectal cancer screening. *Am J Gastroenterol* 1997; **92:** 2171–8.

22. Cockburn J, Thomas RJS, McLaughlin SJ et al, Acceptance of screening for colorectal cancer by flexible sigmoidoscopy. *J Med Screen* 1995; **2:** 79–83.

23. *Weinstein MC, Stason WB, Foundations of cost-effectiveness analysis for health and medical practices. *N Engl J Med* 1977; **296:** 716–21.

24. Brown ML, Knopf KB, Is colorectal cancer screening really cost-effective? *Desk Reference/Prim Care Cancer* 1999; **19:** 15–21.

25. Whynes DK, Neilson AR, Robinson MHE et al, Colorectal cancer screening and quality of life. *Qual Life Res* 1994; **3:** 191–8.

26. Eddy DM, Screening for colorectal cancer. *Ann Intern Med* 1990; **113:** 373–84.

27. Whynes DK, Neilson R, Walker AR et al, Faecal occult blood screening for colorectal cancer: Is it cost-effective? *Health Econ* 1998; **7:** 21–9.

28. Gyrd-Hansen D, Sogaard J, Kronborg O, Colorectal cancer screening: efficiency and effectiveness. *Health Econ* 1998; **7:** 9–20.

29. Loeve F, Brown ML, Boer R et al, Endoscopic colorectal cancer screening: a cost-saving analysis. *J Natl Cancer Inst* 2000; **92:** 557–63.

30. Eddy DM, Screening for cervical cancer. *Ann Intern Med* 1990; **113:** 214–26.

31. Edelson JT, Weinstein MC, Tosteson AN et al, Long-term cost-effectiveness of various initial monotherapies for mild to moderate hypertension. *JAMA* 1990; **263:** 407–13.

32. Goldman L, Weinstein MC, Goldman PA et al, Cost-effectiveness of HMG-CoA reductase inhibition for primary and secondary prevention of coronary heart disease. *JAMA* 1991; **265:** 1145–51.

33. Winawer SJ, St John DJ, Bond JH et al, Prevention of colorectal cancer: guidelines based on new data. *WHO Bulletin OMS* 1995; **73:** 7–10.

34. *U.S. Preventive Services Task Force. Screening for colorectal cancer. In: *Guide to Clinical Preventive Services.* Baltimore: Williams & Wilkins, 1996; 89–103.

35. Colorectal cancer screening, Medicare: http://www.hcfa.gov.news /pr2001/pr010414.htm.

36. Saito H, Yoshida Y, Mass screening: Japanese perspective. In: *Prevention and Early Detection of Colorectal Cancer* (Young GP, Rozen P, Levin B, eds). London: Saunders, 1996; 301–11.

37. The European Group for Colorectal Cancer Screening, Recommendation to include colorectal cancer screening in public health policy. *J Med Screen* 1999; **6:** 80–1.

38. *Rozen P, The OMED Colorectal Cancer Screening Committee: a report of its aims and activities. *Gastrointest Endosc* 1999; **50:** 449–54.

39. Ganiats TG, A spectrum of health policy methods: lessons from the British. *J Fam Pract* 1997; **45:** 391–3.

40. Norum J, Prevention of colorectal cancer: a cost-effectiveness approach to a screening model employing sigmoidoscopy. *Ann Oncol* 1998; **9:** 613–8.

41. Gow J, Costs of screening for colorectal cancer: an Australian programme. *Health Econ* 1999; **8:** 531–40.

42. Members of the National Health Committee Working Party on Population Screening for Colorectal Cancer, Recommendations on population screening for colorectal cancer in New Zealand. *NZ Med J* 1999; **112:** 4–6.

43. The Canadian Task Force on the Periodic Health Examination, Screening for colorectal cancer. In: *The Canadian Guide to Clinical Preventive Health Care* (Solomon M, McLeod R, eds). Ottawa: Canada Communication Group–Publishing, 1994: 797–807.

44. Whynes DK, Cost-effectiveness of faecal occult blood screening for colorectal cancer: results of the Nottingham trial. *Crit Rev Oncol Hematol* 1999; **32:** 155–65.

45. Wright JC, Weinstein MC, Gains in life expectancy from medical interventions – standardizing data on outcomes. *N Engl J Med* 1998; **339:** 380–6.

Index